DR. CAS

Lifesaving CURES

How to use the **latest** and **most** **powerful** natural **cures** for the 21st century

Knowledge House

Buffalo Grove, Illinois

First Edition

Printed in the United States of America on Recycled Paper

Disclaimer: This book is not intended as a substitute for medical
diagnosis or treatment. Anyone who has a serious disease should
consult a physician before initiating any change in treatment or
before beginning any new treatment. Note: the purpose of this
book is to provide vital information in the event of castrophes. It
is not meant as a guide for self-medication or as replacement for
standard medical care. To reiterate, if you suffer from a medical
condition, see your physician.

Ordering information
This book may be ordered from any bookstore by using the title
or ISBN number: 0-911119-99-X. For prompt mail order call:
1-800-243-5242.

To pay by money order enclose $19.95 plus $5.00 S & H to:
Knowledge House P.O. Box 4885 Buffalo Grove, IL 60089.
Add $1.00 postage for each additional book. For orders of 3 to 5
books postage is free. For orders of 6 to12 books the price is
$15.00 each plus postage (as above). Delivery is prompt (within 2 weeks).
For bulk or case orders call: 1-800-243-5242.

TABLE OF CONTENTS

Introduction

The objective of this book is simple. It is to describe what is most effective and easy to use to quickly cure disease. It is to elucidate the most safe natural remedies for a wide range of illnesses. It is to document which substances can be relied upon to improve the odds of survival in the 21st century. It is to prepare the individual for the decades ahead. These decades will certainly deliver health crises of mammoth proportions. The result will be disability, disease, and death beyond our imagination and far exceeding the capacity of modern medicine alone to resolve. Thus, the primary objective is to enable the individual to become capable of self-care through natural cures, which are non-toxic, easy to use, and lifesaving.

Few people know how to take care of themselves in the event of a collapse of personal health let alone a national crisis. Yet, the need for self-help in the health field is greater now than ever before in modern history. This book helps prepare the individual for the potential health consequences of breakdowns in infrastructure in Western countries as well as disease/epidemics. When health disasters strike, the individual must have available natural substances that work quickly, safely, and reliably for reversing common illnesses and injuries.

The need for such remedies is enormous. Billions of humans suffer pain, agony, and distress from potentially curable conditions, and the greatest hope for cure lies in the remedies of nature. This method of using safe/natural remedies to cure disease is based upon the principles of the Hippocratic Oath, to which every physician testifies upon graduating. The medicine of Hippocrates, the supposed father of medicine, was based exclusively on food and herbs.

The health of Americans is declining, largely because of the devastation of the immune system, which results from modern living. Bizarre germs are attacking our bodies, and our immune systems are failing to successfully combat them. In terms of total loss of productivity cold and flu viruses wreak the greatest devastation. Food poisoning epidemics afflict tens of millions yearly and permanently disable thousands. Powerful viruses infect our bodies' organs at will, causing untold misery and/or permanent damage. Ticks are infesting humanity with rodent derived germs from which no drug can protect us. We thought we were well immunized. Yet, whooping cough and diphtheria are returning. Antibiotics were supposed to protect us. Yet, there are thousands of bizarre mutant bacteria, which are immune to antibiotics. In particular, drug resistant staph, strep, Salmonella, and E. coli are causing frightening and often lethal epidemics. Infectious diseases are no longer seasonal; they disrupt our lives on a monthly, weekly, and, in some instances, daily basis.

Natural disasters are also increasing the risks and not just in disaster zones. Epidemics which start in distant regions can spread rapidly, affecting humanity globally. Mass transport has made this a reality. The year of 1998 heralded the greatest disasters of this generation. Over 50,000 people were killed and tens of millions injured and/or displaced by monster disasters. Hurricanes Georges and Mitch, devastating tornadoes in the southwestern USA, massive earthquakes in Afghanistan, Japan, and Columbia, volcanic eruptions in Mexico, the great Yangtze flood, typhoons and tempests in the South Seas, and disastrous forest fires all over the world have destroyed the lives of the people and the ecosystems. Yet, the greatest damage to humanity is forthcoming. As a result of these monstrous disasters, untold thousands more will likely suffer from potentially fatal illnesses. Disaster zones, especially flood zones, breed disease. The decimation in the aftermath will likely be even greater than the original disaster. There is no way to estimate the long term effects, but they will be monumental.

The financial toll is beyond count. The *Chicago Tribune* reported on November 1998, that natural disasters in that year wrought some 90 billion dollars in damage. The editors note that this is more damage than all of the disasters of the past decade, perhaps the past two decades, combined. The massive snow storms of 1999 were another promise of more disastrous events and expenses to come. Thus, it is reasonable to presume that the beginning of the new century will only be worse. This has already been proven in 1999 by the massive Turkish earthquake and the mammoth mile-wide Oklahoma tornado, disasters the likes of which have never been seen in modern history, which occurred just as this book went to press.

In one year, 1998, there were a greater number of severe natural catastrophes than those occurring in the entire decade from 1988 through 1998. What can be expected in the 21st century? Assuredly, at a minimum the same level of destruction is likely. Yet, there will be events in the 21st century delivering destruction of even greater magnitude, a level of human suffering far beyond the 1998 experience. In fact, the degree of destruction, deluge, disease, and despair likely to strike in the 21st century may well be unfathomable. The negative effects of human meddling will inevitably destroy us.

Certain individuals, including so-called experts, might regard this as "doomsday advice." Yet, these are the same individuals who failed to predict, advise, or warn about the potential for disasters such as Hurricane Mitch, which destroyed Nicaragua and Honduras. The destruction of an entire country is unprecedented in modern history. None of these "experts" predicted it. Nor do these individuals warn the public about the disasters of modern medicine: antibiotic resistance, super-germs, mutant viruses, toxic drug reactions, the toxicity and futility of chemotherapy, the excessive use of radiotherapy, the toxicity of margarine, genetically engineered foods, or any of the other preventable "American disasters." Nor did they or would they prepare the populous for toxic chemical or radiation disasters such as those which occurred in Bhopal, Three Mile Island, or Chernobyl. Neither do they warn us of the disastrous effects of daily exposure to poisonous chemicals such as pesticides, herbicides, fungicides, chlorinated hydrocarbons, etc. One wonders what the motives are of those who warn the public not to listen to valuable or lifesaving advice. What would be the motive of covering up or distorting the truth? That is certainly a question worth examining.

Y2K: an *UN*natural Disaster?

Today, North Americans face what is potentially one of the greatest disasters ever. The challenge before each individual is what is the individual to do if the systems to which he/she is accustomed, the technologically based conveniences of modern living, are disrupted? What will the individual do if he/she is cut off from the health care system? Americans have become accustomed to the luxury of having professional health care constantly available. However, the Y2K phenomenon, as well as the potential for massive natural (or unnatural) disasters, eliminates that security. For those who are unfamiliar Y2K signifies a dilemma caused by human error. Computer programmers encoded incomplete information in older computers by listing the year 2000 erroneously as "00." Since computers are mathematical devices, they will be unable to configure this "date." This may result in widespread computer failures as well as destruction of computer files. In fact, the computers will misread the date as 1900 instead of 2000. Thus, they may deliver inaccurate information, which would likely lead to enormous disruptions in commerce, industry, and health care.

Y2K and similar technological errors place every Westerner on the brink, the very population which is least prepared to combat illness/injury, with reliable natural cures. No one knows for sure what will happen as a result of computer outages. What is certain is that there will exist in the United States and Canada a level of chaos never previously experienced. Even the CIA, notoriously silent about issues pertaining to the public, is voicing concern. The agency warns of a "Global Y2K crisis" affecting all sectors of the economy. However, perhaps the most ominous prediction comes from Senator Robert Bennet, head of the U.S. Senate Special Committee on Y2K, who proclaimed the breakdown of computer networks will be one of the most "devastating events" ever to strike America.

Large scale national or international computer crashes have never before occurred in the Western world. It was U.S. Representative Stephen Horn (R-Calif) who stated, "The Year 2000 problem could result in a *stunning array of technological failures* (italics mine)." The *Chicago Tribune* echoes this view, stating that, uncorrected, Y2K will trigger a "vast array of problems." Jaquelyn Williams-Bridges, the State Department's Inspector General for Y2K related issues, testified to a senate subcommittee that "there will be Y2K related failures at every corner of the globe." Furthermore, she stated that health care is the #1 problem and that the level of preparedness is virtually zero. Furthermore, the headline article for the *Chicago Tribune*, Wednesday, March 3rd, 1999, reads "Doctor's offices not ready for Y2K."

If these predictions from highly respected conservative sources prove correct, the individual will be forced to become self-reliant for his/her medical care. Perhaps it won't be as severe as such statements indicate. On the other hand, it might be far worse. The point is when it comes to an individual's health and personal safety, why take chances?

Today, medicine is highly computerized. Technical failures in equipment or systems will compromise the quality of health care. Here is an example of the possibilities. During 1998 a pharmacy chain in Pennsylvania attempted a test on their computers to see if they were Y2K compliant. When the year 2000 was entered into the computer system, the system shut down, and all of the data for thousands of patients was lost. Of even greater concern is the fact that medical machinery is heavily computerized. If critical care devices, such as heart monitors, x-ray machines, and IV pumps, malfunction because of computer chip problems, patients' lives would be put at risk. One authority claims that as a result of the Y2K debacle as many as 6,000 Americans will die in hospitals in the year 2000 as a result of failed medical machinery. Yet, the risk of disease or death in the 21st century from "non-Y2K" disasters is far greater: for instance, epidemics and/or natural disasters.

To rely exclusively on the medical profession for aid in disasters, whether large or small, is potentially disastrous itself. What's more, think of the dilemma posed if the Y2K disaster is combined with a huge natural disaster such as an earthquake or hurricane. No one could be completely prepared for that. The fact is Americans, as well as other

Westerners, such as Canadians and British, are the only individuals who fail completely in having a working knowledge of home remedies. Self care through what may be called home remedies or "self-remedies" must become a 21st century reality. This must happen on a large scale in the American population if individuals are to be assured of proper care and safety in the event of catastrophes.

Think about it. It doesn't require a major disaster for the individual to be forced to rely on home remedies. After all, doctors no longer make house calls and being stranded is a reality despite modern technology. For instance, entire cities, in fact entire states, may be stranded merely by a snow storm or perhaps a flood. In January 1998, an ice storm completely disrupted electricity in Maine, upstate New York, and Canada, cutting power off to thousands of individuals for as long as three weeks. Incredibly, thousands of individuals suffered from cold exposure. Furthermore, as a result of poor quality food and water hundreds contracted infections. Imagine what would happen if a national power outage or some other disruption affecting food/water purity occurred; millions could develop significant infections. On New Year's Day, 1999, a great snow storm struck Chicago, which is inhabited by some 12 million people: few could feasibly reach a physician, and this scenario lasted for several days. What's more, nearly a quarter of a million travelers were stranded at airports and airport hotels throughout the country, some for nearly a week. There is no doubt that the flu bug attacked a larger than normal percentage of this group of highly stressed, agitated, and immune compromised individuals. Yet, none of these displaced people had anywhere to turn for help. The fact is medical personnel themselves were victims of the weather, and there was no guarantee of receiving emergency aid.

As this book went to press the world was stricken with massive disasters: earthquakes, tidal waves, deluge, epidemics, and toxic contamination. In a mere 60 days monstrous earthquakes struck Turkey and Taiwan; Typhoon Bart pummelled Okinawa; Hurricaine Floyd destroyed eastern North Carolina: epidemics loom as a result. None of this is by chance.

Everyone has his/her own disaster story to tell. Think about how much more secure such individuals would feel if they developed a working knowledge of natural/home remedies and, more importantly, if they had such remedies on hand. If it is merely stress, upset schedules, and a lack of sleep that are the sole consequences, the individual will recover and life will quickly return to normal; the home remedies might never be administered. However, if such a circumstance is combined with a health disaster, whether it be a horrible bout of the flu, a cold, an earache (which is particularly disastrous when flying, causing perhaps further delay), severe pain, or perhaps something worse, it could be devastating. What a disaster this would be, unless a person is prepared. Armed with a thorough knowledge of natural cures the individual would be prepared and could handle virtually any crisis more efficiently. These are remedies that can be packed in any luggage or purse. Many fit merely in a pocket. In such circumstances is there anything else that the populous could rely upon?

Natural remedies may be useful for preventing catastrophes that could cost life or limb or which could result in pain or misery. However, the objective herein is not to antiquate emergency medical care. Rather, it is to enhance it, perhaps upgrade it in an area in which it is impotent. Medicine has its critical role. Yet, it fails in providing the public with self care options, which are lifesaving in the event of crisis or disaster. These options are also essential in the event of mass computer chaos, which may develop in the 21st century. However, the tantamount need is for the use of natural cures for everyday illnesses, which cause enormous disability currently. What's more, there is no way that modern medicine will be able to handle the health consequences of a massive disaster due to radiation releases, germ epidemics, or toxic chemical exposure. The individual must assume the responsibility for survival.

To be optimally prepared everyone should comprehend options which are safe and which offer powerful biological activity. This book provides precisely that information. As a result of a thorough study of this book the individual will learn the following to assist in preparing for the precarious future:

1. the most effective self-remedies for infections, *in case the antibiotics fail*
2. the most valuable cures for healing wounds
3. the most powerful substances for producing strength and energy
4. foods which offer the greatest fuel and energy power

5. foods which offer the greatest nutrient density for the money
6. the most effective home remedies for halting or preventing epidemics
7. the most useful anti-pain self-remedies
8. the safest self-remedies for children and the elderly
9. natural cures which do not severely interact with prescription medications
10. the top natural cures for reversing radiation poisoning
11. the top natural cures for reversing toxic chemical damage
12. the best natural cures for combating burns
13. the most effective natural cures for inactivating venomous wounds
14. the top self-remedies for reversing poisoning by prescription medication and other potentially toxic substances, that is poison antidotes that are safe to administer in the field
15. the most efficient self-remedies for sunburn and exposure to the elements
16. the best self-remedies for combating the stress and pressure that occur during difficulties/catastrophes or as a result of injury
17. the most chemical free and natural sources of supplements available
18. supplements which are not derived from genetically engineered plants

A knowledge of natural remedies is essential for guaranteeing the best odds for survival. Certainly, relying upon the typical non-prescription items is virtually useless. In fact, their use may prove dangerous. If there is a health disaster, the worst thing to do is to potentiate it. The dispensation of prescription medications by the general public is totally ill advised. No one should consume these drugs unless under a physician's care. Non-prescription drugs are just as precarious. In fact, basic drugs, such as aspirin, acetaminophen, and ibuprofen, result in thousands of deaths yearly, even through "normal" use. So, if non-prescription medicines, such as aspirin, digestive aids, and topical antibiotics, offer little hope and if prescription medications are too risky to self-consume, what is left? It is the natural cures which contain the power and safety that only nature itself can produce. They alone are the agents which can be relied upon for salvation and survival.

Objections have been raised that no research has been done

with the natural cures, indicating that they may not always be safe. Yet, if you are careful to only buy the best natural unadulterated products, such products would be far safer to consume than non-prescription drugs. The wild food and herb products have been used for centuries with great success, and research verifies this. These wilderness foods/herbs are completely safe for human consumption. In contrast, biologically or chemically altered products present unknown variables and significant problems. Chemically or genetically altered products have no record of safety. In fact, according to recent research their safety is dubious.

All of the survival remedies described in this book are safe, effective, and easy to use. Even children should be taught how to use these lifesaving substances. Disasters create panic, but preparedness can avert further calamity and perhaps needless deaths. Study this information; master it. It could prove lifesaving.

Everyone deserves the right to know about simple life-enhancing emergency procedures. The public must know as much as possible about safe and easy to access remedies, which may be used for health improvement as well as emergencies. The federal government is attempting to restrict free speech, essentially violating the constitution, by blocking the dissemination of valuable information in the field of natural healing. This blockade is largely instigated by special interest groups, especially the pharmaceutical cartel. This cartel is notorious for its attempts to restrict freedom of choice.

Government proposes to be the agent for protecting the public. Yet, it gives the public no audience for informed choice. The information blockade is to the detriment of the general public. While the sale of products is allowed, valuable—and scientific—information about such products is restricted and/or prohibited. What is the reasoning behind the policy to allow a product to be sold and yet disallow information? It is, in fact, a dangerous method. Indeed, information would allow the individual to make an intelligent choice and would assist in the proper use of a product and to determine what is helpful or harmful. It is the lack of information that is potentially damaging. It was David Kessler, M.D., then acting FDA Commissioner, who expressed on national TV the government's position, saying, essentially, 'trust us, you mindless idiots, we will make the decisions for you.'

CHAPTER 1

It Will Happen

There will be epidemics of mammoth proportions in the 21st century. The world's leading scientists share this viewpoint. It was Dr. J. Lederberg, Nobel Prize winner and current President of Rockefeller University, who said that the threat of a massive epidemic sweeping the Western world is "real...and looming." Virtually no one will be completely prepared. Lederberg states that there is no way that the government will be prepared and that the hospitals are ill equipped and will be "absolutely swamped."

The epidemics of the 21st century will involve a wide range of germs and a massive number of people. Virtually every country will be affected. No one will be prepared completely. Yet, a thorough knowledge of self-remedies and natural cures will place the informed in an elite, perhaps enviable, position.

There should be great concern about the issue of massive epidemics. Concern is protective, because it creates action. In contrast, inaction, the bane of modern humanity, is deadly. Don't be reticent. You yourself might be one of the unfortunate statistics if you fail to develop a knowledge of what you can do to protect yourself, your loved ones, and perhaps a total stranger.

AIDS is a global epidemic. So is hepatitis. Fungal infections are the bugaboo of Western societies, and infections by an extensive range of fungi, including Candida albicans, are widespread. Drug resistant microbes—strep, staph, E. coli, Salmonella, and others—are decimating the population, afflicting tens of millions of individuals. The *JAMA* (*Journal of American Medical Association*) noted in 1997 that antibiotic resistant germs kill on a yearly basis a minimum of 250,000 hospitalized patients alone. Thus, epidemics already exist. However, these epidemics will worsen as the 21st century progresses. Be prepared so you can protect yourself. If you become the victim, you can't even help yourself let alone anyone else. What's more, if you fall ill, there may be no one to come to your aid.

Can you imagine the consequences of epidemics of such a massive scale that tens of millions of individuals will become infected? Microbiologists insist such a scenario is inevitable. They claim it is a natural cycle of human civilization. Yet, epidemics are current in America. This is largely because chronic infections by mutant germs afflict tens of millions of Americans. In 1999 a bizarre flu-like illness struck millions, the flu shot seemingly offering little if any protection. Instead of lasting the typical week or so, symptoms persisted as long as six weeks, severely weakening infected individuals. Yet, it was Dr. Lederberg who described the return of the cycle of epidemic infection, not nationally but, rather, globally. He predicts that a pandemic, that is a global epidemic afflicting untold millions, perhaps billions, will strike at any moment. His view is shared by the majority of microbiologists.

The viruses of the current era are highly invasive. Nothing in the medical system can stop them. They are bizarre, mutated, and, thus, incredibly dangerous. It is not a matter of if they will strike or even when—they are already here.

Judy Kay Gray, M.S., research scientist, describes the following frightening scenario: "Global warming is the incubator for the newest wave of infectious diseases; warmth breeds germs. The melting of the icebergs is releasing vast numbers of germs frozen in time for thousands of years. Along with the mutations of virulent germs already in existence, we are being exposed to killer pathogens previously not encountered by the current generation. This enormous germ burden will inundate the global population, which has no immunity to these freakish germs. The result will be disease, disability, and death at levels never before previously experienced."

The new millennium will be fraught with uncountable disasters, both naturally and humanly induced, causing an unprecedented degree of strife and suffering. The fact is such human despair is currently happening, for instance, disease outbreaks in Honduras and Nicaragua, the tropical diseases infesting the Chinese as a result of the Yangtze flood, and the millions of North Americans suffering from chronic infections due to antibiotic resistant germs.

There is particular concern about the global consequences of the great 1999 natural disasters. The enormous numbers of individuals displaced by natural disasters validates this prediction. Displacement consequently results in disease. The masses are crowded virtually upon each other with nowhere to live, eat, breathe, sleep, or hide. In this setting of strife, stress, and poor nutrition, communicable diseases spread rapidly. In other words, the germs will spread like a wild fire. As a result, rampant epidemics will strike humanity, and the loss in lives could be in the millions, perhaps tens of millions. For instance, in China in 1998 a world record flood occurred along the Yangtze River, displacing over 20 million people. What's more, the flood occurred, from the point of view of the spread of infectious disease, at the worst possible time: the summer, which aids in the breeding of germs. This may lead to local, as well as international, epidemics. The Chinese population, as well as the animals of China, harbor a wide variety of germs, notably influenza viruses and parasites. These germs are notorious for causing epidemics. Recall the Swine Flu concerns of the 1970s as well as the more current Hong Kong and "chicken" flu syndrome. Mexico/Central America is another hot zone for the spread of infection. In Central America Hurricane Mitch forced tens of thousands from their homes, immediately resulting in outbreaks of dengue fever, malaria, influenza, cholera, and fungal infections. For instance, in March, 1999, an encephalitis epidemic struck Malaysia, leading to over 120 deaths. Most of the deaths occurred in pork farmers/processors, and, in fact, the virus was proven to be transmitted from swine to humans. No medicine could be found to halt the infection. The Malaysian government resorted to the slaughter of tens of thousands of pigs in an attempt to control the epidemic. The point is that if this virus had invaded the population at large potentially thousands of humans would have been killed. The Malaysian experience proves that such catastrophes are highly likely to occur in the future.

Throughout the United States floods have accelerated the growth of bizarre fungi and molds capable of decimating health. Potentially millions of individuals are developing illnesses from these highly toxic molds. In the Ohio and Mississippi river valleys hundreds of thousands of individuals are sickened by the highly poisonous mold chemicals known as mycotoxins: many die.

Yet, the majority of illnesses are unrelated to acts of nature. They are happening to individuals in daily life. An example of this is the disaster of a health care worker who contracts AIDS or hepatitis or perhaps some unknown infection from human contaminants. Other examples include the crisis of a surgical patient, who develops a bizarre drug resistant infection which is more dangerous than the surgical issue and the individual whose organs are attacked by a virus or bacteria after receiving tainted blood. There is also the individual who contracts a disastrous internal infection from merely eating commercial, but tainted, food. These are the disasters of everyday life that account for a greater degree of disability, pain, and anguish than any other factor.

Medical mishaps increase the risks for global epidemics as well as local crises. The overuse of antibiotics in hospitals has led to thousands of outbreaks of infections, which are virtually impossible to halt with even the most potent of all medicines. Tens of thousands of deaths have been attributed to these drug-induced outbreaks. Research labs carelessly release test germs, which may populate the environment, leading to potentially bizarre diseases. Genetic engineering leads to the introduction of unknown proteins in food and vegetation, which will likely cause new illnesses and severe allergic reactions. In what is acclaimed as "science for the future of humankind" chicken, bacterial, and fish genes are added to vegetables. This fabrication would never develop in nature. The potential damage in humans from such fabrications has never been carefully assessed. Yet, with nearly 50% of all modern food containing genetically engineered components, soon the effects of this "experiment" will surface. Far from being scientific or altruistic, this is a global commercial movement, which has exclusively financial motivations. It is to the detriment of the human race, as well as the world's precious array of animals and plants, to alter the gene pool in an invasive, unnatural way.

Modern medicine is largely technology driven, which could prove disastrous in the event of man-made errors such as the year 2000 issue. According to Dr. Donald Palmisano, an AMA board member, computer errors can be deadly. While testifying before the Senate's Y2K subcommittee, he described a hospital horror story. Three patients were killed as a result of a malfunctioning radiation machine, which delivered massive doses because of a computer error, one that was not Y2K related.

Already, nearly half of all deaths globally are attributed to infections. Even with cancer, the majority of deaths are due to infectious complications, such as pneumonia, blood poisoning, kidney infections, etc., rather than any direct effects of the tumors. Hostile germs and drug-resistant bacteria are currently the cause of unmitigated global crises. Invasive medical procedures, as well as potent medications, are responsible for additional damage and disease, particularly in the Western world. Since there is already chaos, any breakdown in the status quo and/or infrastructure will accentuate the danger. The result will be an increased incidence of life-threatening illnesses, that is a global health crisis.

In the 21st century Westerners will be at a high risk for natural and man-made disasters. Aging infrastructure, human error, and natural catastrophes all contribute to this risk. Sabotage, while admittedly a risk, is insignificant comparatively. The following is a listing of potential dangers to acknowledge and prepare for:

1. chemical and radioactive pollution
2. lack of potable water
3. inadequate clean, safe, nutritious food
4. rampant infections from highly invasive germs
5. inadequate protection from the elements, i.e. too hot or too cold, with no means of mitigating it (power outages, disaster-induced loss of shelter, etc.)
6. lack of sewage disposal and garbage disposal
7. violent tendencies of individuals, especially those who are totally unprepared for disasters, technology breakdowns, etc.
8. angry hostile individuals who take out their stress on others.

CHAPTER 2

The Cures

If your options are compromised and you are forced to abandon everything, don't forget to grab your home remedies. It is these remedies that will make the difference between survival and disaster. This book helps you select items which are easy to use and readily available. Lack of toxicity is crucial in these scenarios, and, thus, virtually all of the remedies described herein are non-toxic. In other words, they cannot kill you or hurt your organs. In fact, the only significant effect of these natural substances is positive. In other words, they will help you get well and will possibly save your life and perhaps the lives of those you encounter.

Aloe vera

Since 3000 B.C. aloe vera has been used as an emergency medicine. Aloe is versatile, because it speeds the healing of wounds, plus it kills germs. However, its main use in wound healing is for sunburn. Aloe is always helpful for this condition. It induces healing, prevents scarring, and helps cool the body. Thus, it is a most useful agent to apply in the event of heat exhaustion and sunburn. Aloe, straight from the plant, is also useful for any type of skin irritation. What's more, research performed in Chicago indicates that aloe may offer another anti-burn action: frostbite.

17

Dr. M. Robson, a surgeon, discovered that aloe taken directly from the plant and added to a skin cream outright cured frostbite, preventing amputation in serious frostbite cases. Other uses of aloe include healing of chemical burns, steam burns, cold sores, canker sores, swollen/sore gums, open wounds, and skin cancer.

Bee propolis

Bee propolis is the bees' favorite antibiotic. Bees collect a substance from the buds of trees resembling a type of resin. They convert the resin to propolis. A flavonoid-rich substance, propolis exhibits both antiinflammatory and antiseptic properties. It is also an anti-toxin, helping to reverse or protect against toxic chemical and/or radiation exposure.

Propolis is defined in Webster's dictionary as "bee glue." Indeed, despite its valuable anti-germ properties bees use it primarily as a glue for cementing their hives. Yet, it serves a dual function, because it is a germ resistant coating. Bees use propolis to prevent germ infestation in the hive by carefully coating the entire surface, internally as well as externally, with this precious substance. The power of propolis in this respect is evident to anyone who sees an abandoned hive; the hive remains intact for years or, perhaps, decades without visible decay. Bees also use propolis to coat foreign objects which gain entry to their hives. Astonishingly, a mouse was once found in a bee hive. After stinging it to death, the bees coated it with propolis. Incredibly, the propolis coating preserved the mouse virtually intact, mummifying it. In other words, it halted all microbial actions. Obviously, propolis is a natural preservative. The reliance upon it also explains why thousands of bees can live in tight quarters without the risk of devastating epidemics.

Propolis is one of nature's most unique antibiotics, offering germ killing powers against virtually any organism, particularly viruses, bacteria, fungi, and parasites. In contrast to prescription antibiotics germs are unable to develop resistance to it. Furthermore, it is safe to self-administer during a crisis both topically and internally. Propolis is non-toxic, that is as long as it is pure and free of pollutants. The problem is that propolis may contain lead. The lead is not from pollution. It is from the beehives, that is man-made hives. The hives are painted, often with lead based paint. When the propolis, which the bees glue to the hives, is scraped off, paint is removed along with it. Propolis is so sticky that there is no way to remove the paint. Thus, when the propolis is processed, lead and other chemicals from the paint are perilously intermixed. When buying propolis, be sure it is assayed and proven lead-free. The importance of guaranteed lead free sources is aptly illustrated by the following:

Case history: A 45 year-old woman aggressively used bee propolis for a severe gum infection. Buying a standard brand of propolis tincture, she consumed as much as one-half ounce per day. Within a week, she developed visual changes, fatigue, nausea, and blinding headaches. A complete blood count was performed. Tests revealed an abnormality known as *basophillic stippling*, which is a classic marker for lead poisoning. Thus, this patient developed acute lead poisoning from contaminated propolis. After halting the propolis, the symptoms eventually diminished.

Black seed (Nigella seed)

It was the brilliant Prophet Muhammad who said that Nigella seed could potentially cure nearly any disease. This seed is a native of the Mediterranean and African regions and has been used as food and medicine for thousands of years. Found in the Pharoahs' tombs, it was renowned in numerous ancient Mediterranean civilizations for its health giving properties. The Greeks and Romans regarded it as one of their top medicinal herbs. Dioscorides (1st century A.D.) gave dozens of uses for it. Nigella, he claimed, eradicated headaches, sinus problems, toothaches, menstrual disorders, and intestinal parasites. Today, its antiparasitic actions are perhaps most renowned. African/Asian herbalists use it to purge the bowel of worms, especially in children. It is also relied upon for reversing gas, stomach ache, and intestinal cramps. In India it is taken extensively to enhance breast milk formation and is perhaps the most effective herb known for this purpose. I have personally found it effective for curtailing the devastating symptoms of the flu.

Modern research confirms black seed's significant therapeutic properties. Egyptian physicians determined that black seed reversed asthma better than common medications. Other studies point to the spice's immune boosting powers. Apparently, it is one of the most powerful immune enhancing agents known.

Nigella seed is exceptionally pungent. This is what accounts for its medicinal properties. It is very rich in natural oils, which nourish and soothe the body. The highly aromatic components warm the tissues, stimulate digestion, and activate metabolism. Thus, it is a tonic valuable for nearly all ailments.

Bromelain

Enzymes are the most powerful living force of the body. They are the body's workhorses, performing thousands of essential functions.

Bromelain is an extremely useful enzyme, and it was selected for this book because of its versatility and potency. It is a protein digesting enzyme extracted from pineapples, not the fruit but the green stem.

Bromelain is one of the most reliable tissue healing agents known. It aids in the healing of any injury. It does so by stimulating circulation and by eliminating swelling and inflammation.

Only uncoated bromelain, the type found in capsules, is reliable as a supplement. The best bromelain is certified by assay to digest protein in an activity against milk protein, i.e. milk clotting units (MCU), or against gelatin, i.e. gelatin dissolving units (GDU). Never purchase enteric coated or hard tablet bromelain. These tablets are ineffective compared to the uncoated variety.

A typical dosage for combating trauma is 2 to 4 capsules taken on an empty stomach several times daily. A high grade product measures a minimum of 400,000 MCU, that is Milk Clotting Units, or 2000 GDU (Gelatin Dissolving Units) per 1000 mg. Continue this dosage until improvement is noted. Then, reduce the amount to 1 or 2 capsules twice daily. Papain, the protein digesting enzyme from papayas, is synergistic with bromelain. This enzyme is measured both in Milk Clotting Units and Proteolytic Units. Ideally, a top quality product should contain both enzymes. The papain should measure a minimum of 1000 MCU or 25,000 Proteolytic Units per 1000 mg.

Don't expect pineapples to provide enough bromelain to exert a physiological effect. The enzyme is concentrated in the green stems, not the fruit, although fresh pineapple contains a greater amount than the canned. Papaya fruit contains a considerable amount of papain, however, the highest concentration is found in the seeds. The more green a papaya is the richer it is in enzymes.

Chlorella

Chlorella is one of the most versatile of all emergency remedies. Its versatility is largely because it binds toxic chemicals, removing them from the body. It also helps the body detoxify pesticides and herbicides as well as chlorinated hydrocarbons.

Research proves that chlorella can save lives in the event of any type of disaster, especially toxic chemical and radiation exposure. It can also be taken on a daily basis as a preventive.

Another benefit of chlorella is that it is pure protein. The type of protein it contains is complete and is readily digested into a usable form. Thus, it serves as a source of daily, as well as emergency, nourishment. However, its greatest utility is in the event of chemical poisoning, heavy metal exposure, cyanide poisoning, toxic smoke exposure, etc. Take a large amount of capsules or packets until the symptoms of poisoning improve. This is safe to take in large quantities, because it is essentially a food rather than a medicine. Chlorella taken with Nutri-Sense (see page 70) can sustain life for a prolonged time if necessary.

Cilantro/coriander oil

This is one of the most fascinating of all herbal oils. It was Prophet Muhammad who apparently stated that with the exception of cancer, the cilantro/coriander plant could, if taken regularly, cure virtually any disease. Both cilantro and coriander are fine tonics for the gut. They stimulate digestion and aid in elimination. They are excellent warming agents, meaning they help increase metabolic rate. Today, herbalists use cilantro/coriander for reversing nausea, diarrhea in children, intestinal cramps, stomachache, and hemorrhoids. It is also used for nerve disorders, including migraines, neuralgia, liver disorders, heart disease, and stress syndromes. The latest research edifies its importance for liver function, particularly coriander. This spice greatly enhances the liver's ability to metabolize cholesterol, aiding in bile synthesis and reducing blood cholesterol levels. This may explain why individuals who regularly consume this spice have a reduced incidence of liver problems as well as heart disease.

The best cilantro comes from the Mediterranean, where it grows wild. Here, the cilantro is derived from the green shoots of the coriander plant. The cilantro typically used in recipes, that is the fresh type, isn't from the coriander tops. It is an entirely different plant of Central American origin. North American Herb & Spice Co. provides an oil of cilantro plus coriander made from the actual tops and seeds of the coriander plant. Thus, it is a true oil of cilantro, that is the type used since ancient times as a medicine. Incidentally, this is an exotic food additive and may be used to enliven virtually any recipe, especially meat and poultry dishes. For the latter it acts as a mild antiseptic as well as a preservative.

Cinnamon

This is one of the most ancient of all spices. Historically, it was used both as a medicine and flavoring. Blair's *Biblical Herbal* describes how cinnamon was more valued in ancient Rome than gold. He further mentions how it was relied upon to aid digestion and cure diarrhea.

According to Lee Broadhurst, Ph.D., herbal researcher, cinnamon exhibits significant anti-diabetic action. However, to achieve an anti-diabetic effect significant amounts must be consumed, like a teaspoon or two per day.

Cinnamon is a top spice for survival, plus it is easy to store and virtually impervious to spoilage. Do not use commercial or aromatherapy grade cinnamon oil, which is made from the leaves instead of the edible bark. Use instead the regular commercial spice, or, preferably, freshly ground cinnamon sticks (which may be processed in a coffee grinder). Or, take edible cinnamon oil. This type of oil is made only from the unprocessed natural cinnamon bark, the same type used for the spice. Avoid aromatherapy cinnamon oils. These are usually produced from the leaves and/or root bark, both of which are unfit for human consumption. According to research published by Jean Valnet, a French medical doctor and famous essential oil researcher, edible oil of cinnamon is capable of killing most germs. In a concentration of less than one percent cinnamon oil sterilized septic water.

Cranberries
The main value of cranberries is in the prevention or reversal of urinary tract infections. Thus, they should be utilized primarily by individuals vulnerable to these infections. They are an excellent tonic for the kidneys.

Researchers have thoroughly proven that cranberry juice, as well as the extract in capsules, is highly beneficial in preventing bacteria from attacking the urinary tract. It does so by blocking the ability of the germs to attach to the mucous membranes of these organs. Thus, the microbes are simply flushed out before they can infect the tissues. Only a few berries possess this action, and they all belong to the cranberry family. The active components within these berries are called tannins, also known as proanthocyanidins.

Cranberry Juice
Commercial cranberry juice is not a lifesaving food. It is high in sugar and/or corn syrup. Cranberry concentrate is the ideal type to utilize. It can be readily reconstituted simply by adding water and is free of sugar and additives.

Cranberry is a tart berry, and this is why it is so useful as a health aid. The sour taste is due to a group of compounds known as organic acids. These acids include gallic, in which it is most rich, and malic acid. These organic acids are actually types of flavonoids.

A recent article published in *Life Science* by Dr. T. Wilson shows that cranberry extract is highly beneficial to the heart and circulation. Plus, because of the anti-germ effects of the cranberry acids, it is highly useful in the prevention and treatment of urinary tract disorders, including bladder, prostate, and kidney infections.

Cumin

While it is one of the most relied upon of all herbs in antiquity, cumin is relatively unknown in America. Yet, if ancient tradition is correct, it is another spice worth its weight in gold. This is because this highly pungent spice is a potent natural medicine. Unfortunately, today it is only used in veterinary medicine. Yet, its utility for humans is immense, especially for disorders of the gut.

Most Americans realize how pungent and aromatic oil of cumin is, especially Mexican food lovers. Yet, that is why it is such a valuable substance. Its aroma is due to its high content of special substances known as aldehydes. Specifically, cumin is rich in cuminaldhehyde, and that is what gives it its medicinal power.

Cumin has been used medicinally for thousands of years and was a favorite natural remedy of the ancients; it is mentioned at least twice in the Bible. Mathias notes in *Economic Botany* that this spice has been used as food and medicine since "earliest written records." Apparently, the ancients administered it primarily for digestive and circulatory disorders as well as for headaches. Now it is known that cumin and, particularly, oil of cumin, is one of the most powerful of all antioxidants. When researchers matched oil of cumin against a variety of antioxidants, it showed supremacy over all of them. Cumin oil greatly enhanced the ability of the body to fight toxicity by increasing the synthesis of a critical enzyme called glutathione peroxidase. One study found that as a result of enhanced glutathione activity the ability of organs to remove toxic compounds was increased by up to 700%.

As mentioned, since antiquity cumin has been respected as a digestive aid. Now we know that this effect is due to its valuable actions on the digestive organs, particularly the liver and pancreas.

One study found that oil of cumin increased the liver's output of bile, which is critical for the digestion of fat, by as much as 300%. That is an enormous increase. Another study found that cumin preserves and enhances the function of the pancreas. Cumin also possesses significant antiseptic actions. In particular, it was found to be highly effective in destroying the larvae and eggs of parasites. Yet, cumin is one of the few natural substances possessing potent actions against a wide range of microbes, including worms, protozoans, amoebas, bacteria, and fungi. Furthermore, of all spices tested cumin was one of the few capable of preventing one of the most pervasive of all health issues: food spoilage. The crude essential oil of cumin thoroughly halted the production of dangerous compounds secreted into food by mold/fungi known as *mycotoxins*. What's more, as reported in the *Journal of Food Science*, cumin is an aggressive antifungal agent, which completely inhibited fungal growth in even tiny amounts. Lastly, it is an anti-toxin, meaning it aids the body in the removal of toxic chemicals.

Oil of cumin is extremely pungent, so start by using a small amount, like 2 or 3 drops twice daily. Ideally, add it to tomato/V-8 juice or fatty foods. Then, increase the amount to as much as 20 drops twice daily. Fill a gelatin capsule with the oil for easy administration. Stools tend to become a normal rich dark color, which is an excellent effect and is due to improved bile flow. Because of its dramatic actions in purging the liver of bile, this is one of the most valuable antidotes to poisonous chemicals known.

LivaClenz™ is a special blend of edible plant essential oils containing cumin oil as an active ingredient. It is designed specifically for assisting liver function as well as for detoxification. It contains the oils of a variety of mountain-grown spices, including cumin, fennel, rosemary, and oregano oils. All of these oils have been proven in scientific research to aid in bile production. As a general tonic and preventive agent take 5 drops twice daily. For reversal of mass exposure to toxic chemicals take 20 or more drops three times daily. Both oil of cumin and LivaClenz are useful in assisting liver function. **Note**: the use of an edible extra virgin olive oil emulsion for edible oils was invented by North American Herb & Spice Co. This is the ideal means for the consumption of dietary spice oils.

Fennel

Fennel is the herb which Grecian marathon runners traditionally consumed to give them physical strength and endurance. It has a history as a medicine as ancient as human society itself.

Today, primitives depend upon fennel for treating a number of diseases. In the Middle East it is respected as a dependable tonic for virtually any digestive problem, especially gas and bloating. The ancient Greeks deemed it invaluable for improving vision and increasing life span. It was also used to stimulate weight loss and is apparently very effective for this purpose. This may be explained partially by the fact that fennel, particularly its essential oil, is an aggressive diuretic, speeding the elimination of excess fluid. Fennel is also an excellent aid to liver function. Researchers determined that oil of fennel dramatically increased the output of bile, more than doubling it. In the Mediterranean it is utilized as a gallbladder/liver tonic. It is also respected as a breast tonic. In fact, researchers have proven that oil of fennel dramatically increases breast milk synthesis.

Fennel contains a variety of substances offering natural hormone-like actions. This explains its prolonged use by societies as an aid to female health. Thus, it has been used for menstrual difficulties, bloating, ovarian disorders, and hot flashes. It is far safer as a menopausal aid than synthetic or commercial estrogens.

Care must be taken in the consumption of fennel oil. It is safe, as long as it is derived from the edible seed. The finest fennel comes from its native regions, for instance the Middle East. In contrast, European, American, or South American fennel oil is of inferior quality. An edible Middle Eastern oil of fennel of the highest quality is available from North American Herb & Spice. Be sure that the oil is certified edible before consuming it.

Folic acid

One of the most important of all vitamins, folic acid is critical for the function of every cell in the body. In particular, it is required by the body's DNA repair systems. In other words, when DNA—the genetic material—is damaged (i.e. broken), a process which afflicts each individual daily, folic acid stimulates the repair. The critical importance of this nutrient is edified by the recent reversal of the government posture regarding its daily requirement. The RDA (now known as the RDI) has been nearly tripled, from 150 to 400 mcg per day.

For nearly 50 years the medical profession and U. S. government underestimated the value of this vitamin, even discouraging individuals from consuming large amounts. This was to the detriment of the population. Physicians simply prohibited the consumption of large amounts of this vitamin, that is over 800 micrograms (twice the RDI) per day. They were in error. In fact, their anti-folic acid stance caused significant harm. For instance, tens of thousands of birth defects, ranging from spina bifida and cerebral palsy to cleft palate, could have been prevented through the daily intake of one or more milligrams of folic acid. A recent study proves the degree of error perpetrated by the U. S. government and the medical profession, as well as the pharmaceutical houses, regarding folate intake. Dr. R. A. Jacobs, publishing in the *Journal of Nutrition*, found that in order to halt or prevent DNA damage, the minimum daily intake should be approximately 500 mcg, that is over three times the "old" RDA. When Jacobs gave this amount of folic acid to volunteers, their DNA repair *returned to normal*. Yet, recent reports indicate that for optimal protection even larger amounts may be needed, as much as 5 mg daily.

The minimum of 5 milligrams seems to be the magic dose. A study by Dr. Michel Leeka of Free University Hospital in The Netherlands found that this amount helped completely reverse the damage due to folic acid deficiency. Folic acid deficiency has been associated with a wide range of diseases, including heart disease, cancer, hardening of the arteries, malabsorption syndrome, irritable bowel, and birth defects. The fact is virtually all of these diseases could be prevented—perhaps cured—by the regular intake of large amounts of this vitamin.

What is perhaps even more absurd is the fact that cancer patients have been prohibited from taking folic acid. The presumption is that this vitamin somehow stimulates the growth of cancer cells. This is utterly false, as is proven by the latest research, which clearly shows that cancer is caused by a deficiency of this nutrient. The vitamin is needed for the growth of normal healthy cells, including white blood cells, which protect the body from cellular degeneration. It is required for the synthesis of DNA, the genetic material which governs the repair of cellular structure and the growth of healthy tissue.

The DNA within our bodies is being assaulted on a large scale, especially in the chemically polluted Western world. Plus, Westerners suffer virtual epidemics of diseases directly related to folic acid deficiency. Thus, for such individuals folic acid supplementation is a must.

Garlic

A crisp knowledge of the health benefits of garlic will always prove handy. This is because it is one of the most safe and versatile of all medicinal herbs. Researchers have proven that garlic is enormously valuable for combating a wide range of illnesses. In other words, it is one of those rare substances that is a universal tonic. This means it provides a certain degree of protection for virtually any illness.

Researchers have discovered that garlic is a natural germicide, capable of killing nearly any microbe. Bacteria, parasites, viruses, and fungi all wilt under its powers. It was even found capable of killing the notoriously difficult to eradicate skin fungi, the type that causes athlete's foot. Thus, garlic is universally valuable as a home remedy. It is versatile, available, and inexpensive. It offers anti-toxin, anti-bacterial, anti-viral, anti-fungal, anti-parasitic, and anti-venom powers. It boosts immunity, increases blood flow, stimulates digestion, purges the liver, and strengthens the heart. All of these actions have been thoroughly documented by modern science.

Here is a simple tip that everyone can apply in the event of a crisis. If medical care is unavailable and a serious infection develops, for instance, in a wound or on the skin, what could be procured virtually anywhere on this earth that would sterilize the wound, eliminate the pain, or neutralize the venom? It is reasonable to presume that garlic could be purchased anywhere. Simply crush a few dozen cloves of garlic to remove a few teaspoons of juice. Add the juice to a body or face cream. Apply this mixture to wounds, abrasions, lacerations, burns, venomous bites, or any other infected or inflamed lesions. Note: a significant stinging sensation may occur.

Glutathione

Glutathione is perhaps the most important protein/enzyme compound of the human body. It is the primary molecular tool for protecting the body against the assaults of living: poisons, aging, stress, and poor diet. It is the number one substance for detoxifying chemicals such as heavy metals, radiation, hydrocarbons, pesticides/herbicides, food additives, and other noxious compounds.

There are dozens of types of glutathione molecules in the body. Glutathione peroxidase, its enzyme form, is the most potent type. This enzyme is protected by certain nutrients, notably riboflavin, vitamin C, and vitamin E. Thus, these vitamins are crucial for maintaining glutathione at the highest biological activity and levels for the purpose of the detoxification of poisons.

Glutathione is a relatively simple molecule, so it can be readily produced by the body. However, it is also quickly depleted, especially if the individual is under a great deal of stress, suffering from a chronic disease, or is exposed regularly to toxic chemicals. In the vitamin/mineral kingdom the most important glutathione boosters are vitamin E, selenium, riboflavin, and vitamin C. Herbs/spices that boost glutathione levels include cumin, oregano, rosemary, and sage. Other herbs, such as silymarin or turmeric, are helpful, however, the aforementioned are the most aggressive and powerful. For instance, one study found that cumin oil alone increased tissue glutathione levels by nearly 700%, while rosemary boosted it by some 400%. Taking glutathione-boosting vitamins along with the herbs/spices dramatically improves the operations of the internal glutathione factories, giving the individual ideal health as well as the best chances for combating a deadly disease or toxic crisis.

Honey, unprocessed

This is the ideal substance for combating crisis and illness, because it is both food and medicine. Honey is perhaps humanity's original medicinal food, being utilized for at least 60,000 years. All ancient civilizations relied upon it for nourishment as well as for combating disease.

Honey is a predigested food. This means it is readily digested by virtually anyone. Cane sugar or molasses requires energy to digest; honey requires none. Thus, it helps produce energy. Contrary to popular belief, crude raw honey is well tolerated by infants and is entirely safe for their consumption.

Certain medical doctors prohibit the consumption of honey in infants. In fact, the medical profession has made this policy prevalent in the United States and Canada, but it is not a prevalent attitude in all Westernized countries such as those in Europe or Asia. The honey condemnation arises from the same medical profession which taught mothers to place infants face down for sleeping, a policy which led to the death of countless thousands of infants from sudden death syndrome. Using fear tactics instead of science, today's physicians prohibit the consumption of a totally natural food, which could only aid infant health. There is no increased risk for illness or botulism in infants who are fed raw honey. It is harmless. Rather, the consumption of this natural antiseptic food protects infants from such diseases. The fact is when this substance is placed on wounds infected by the botulism organism, it sterilizes them. Raw honey has been consumed by the primitives and their children for thousands of years. It never has and never will cause botulism. We feed our infants and children all manner of poisons: drugs, antibiotics, sugar water, soda pop, candy, sugary cereals, and deep fried foods, not to speak of the toxic food additives found in virtually all processed foods. Yet, we never worry about any ill effects. One dose of chicken nuggets, bologna, or a can of soda pop should be a source of far greater concern for causing ill health than a spoon of crude raw honey, which mothers in the United States and Canada have stringently avoided giving their children for decades on the basis that it could somehow cause fatal disease. How ludicrous is such thinking.

Raw honey kills germs of all types. A study performed in England found that wounds infected by a variety of germs were sterilized within a few days as a result of the honey applications. The *Journal of Pediatrics* found that honey, even the commercial variety, worked better than the typical pediatric remedies in halting infantile diarrhea. Currently, British surgeons use it on burns with great success. They note that the honey sterilizes the wounds and halts scarring. Here are just a few of the immense uses of honey against disease:

- for halting diarrhea and intestinal cramps
- for preventing infection and scarring in burns
- for firming up sloppy stools (especially in infants)
- for healing wounds and killing germs in wounds
- for application to abrasions, cuts, and sores
- for easing constipation
- for halting coughs and lung congestion
- for aiding in the growth of natural/healthy intestinal bacteria

Kelp

A rich source of iodine and other trace minerals, kelp is one of the most nutrient dense of all food supplements. It is the best naturally occurring source of iodine, which is sorely needed for the function of the glands, particularly the thyroid gland.

Kelp's greatest use is to regenerate the thyroid gland. It greatly balances it, often singlehandedly bringing its function to normal. Tens of millions of Americans, particularly women, suffer from abnormally functioning thyroid glands. Whether the thyroid gland is overactive or underactive, kelp is always effective, because it serves to normalize thyroid function.

Its actions on the thyroid gland also explains its enormous value for disasters. Radiation poisons the thyroid gland. This is the first internal organ to be damaged as a result of a radiation accident. Radioactive iodine is rapidly absorbed into the body, and the thyroid gland vigorously traps all iodine molecules, so if it is exposed to the radioactive type, it doesn't differentiate. Thus, it unwittingly destroys itself. The secret to preventing this is to bombard the thyroid with as much natural iodine as possible to block the entry of the poisonous type. This is utterly crucial. Doing so will prevent cancer and save lives, especially if a nuclear power plant explodes or if some similar radiation disaster occurs. Other forms of iodine should be consumed such as potassium iodide. If a nuclear disaster occurs, overload the body with iodine in the form of kelp, potassium iodide, iodized salt, and crude unbleached sea salt. This one step may save your life.

Warning: there are many inferior types of kelp. They are inferior, because they are harvested from pollution zones. Researchers have discovered that commercial kelp tablets are contaminated with heavy metals. Kelp possesses great affinity for trapping minerals, and it fails to differentiate. It has a particular affinity for arsenic. For instance, several cases of arsenic poisoning have occurred in kelp users. Kelp harvested from remote regions is free of industrial pollutants and is devoid of measurable levels of arsenic or other heavy metals. *PureKelp* by North American Herb & Spice is one such brand. It is assayed and *proven to be free of toxic chemicals, arsenic, or heavy metals*. Before buying kelp be sure to investigate the source. Demand an analysis or procure verbal verification from the maker that it is arsenic/chemical free. Such a pure type of kelp will be a great aid to health, since it is one of the richest sources of nutrients known.

Lactobacillus

There is no question that Lactobacillus bacteria are of value for crisis situations. However, their greatest value is in the prevention or treatment of digestive disorders, particularly diarrhea as well as constipation.

Definitive proof for the power of Lactobacillus came from the University of Nebraska Medical Center. Here, researchers discovered that Lactobacillus was powerful enough to reduce antibiotic induced diarrhea by 300%, a highly significant finding. Previously, the researchers determined that regular consumption of these healthy bacteria speeded recovery from viral gastroenteritis. Thus, Lactobacillus is of particular value for children, who are the primary victims of viral diarrhea. What's more, when taken regularly Lactobacillus apparently helps prevent the diarrhea typically contracted when traveling abroad. This may be why residents of the tropics and the Mediterranean, where food/water sanitation is inferior to that in the Western world, regularly consume Lactobacillus rich foods on a daily/weekly basis. I have seen individuals in these regions drink yogurt by the quart every day.

Take a high quality Lactobacillus supplement as an anti-diarrheal defense. There are dozens of Lactobacillus products on the market. However, use your money wisely. Check with the manufacturer to ensure that the potency is guaranteed and/or that research has been performed on the product. For excellent protection against harmful germs take such a product on a daily basis and increase the consumption of Lactobacillus-rich fermented foods.

Lavender oil

Lavender oil is an immense asset for reversing disease and injury, especially in a crisis. It is one of those unique substances that possesses a broad range of activities. This aromatic flower oil has been a requirement for making life more pleasant for thousands of years. In ancient times the sweet smelling lavender was respected more for its medicinal properties than its scent, while today the opposite is true. Thus, modern society is largely ignoring this oil's greatest attribute: its health-giving properties.

During Biblical times extracts of lavender were used for wound healing. In ancient Persia and Greece lavender was applied as a germ killer. In Medieval times it was famous as an antidote for psychological and neurological disorders. During the 18th century it was part of a world renown formula for beautifying skin and assailing skin ailments. Recent research proves that oil of lavender is an invaluable agent for repairing damaged skin. What's more, it has also been proven to aid in the treatment and prevention of a variety of lung diseases. A. Bissas notes in her article *Lavender— The Essential Oil* that currently lavender is successfully used for combating insomnia, tension, water retention, bad breath, sinus congestion, dandruff, and sluggish circulation. This is not mere folklore. Bissas' comments were recently echoed by the prestigious British journal *The Lancet*, which described how fumes from lavender oil induced sleep equally as well as sleeping medications. Lavender's sedative actions are broad spectrum. It is a reliable relaxing agent for virtually any condition associated with stress or tension, and that means practically all illnesses. Europeans currently use it for migraines. Dr. Jean Valnet, the famous French essential oil expert, used lavender oil for healing skin diseases as well as open wounds. Tisserand notes that it exerts a calming action on the heart and nerves as well as the digestive tract. He describes its European use for colic, nausea, vomiting, gas, and heartburn. A highly technical journal has reported that lavender is an anti-cancer agent. Writing in *Cancer Biotechnology Weekly*, the authors provide data indicating that the oil works as well as chemotherapy drugs without side effects. Currently, lavender oil is being researched by a number of universities for its obvious anti-cancer powers against a wide range of conditions, including breast, intestinal, prostate, and ovarian cancers.

Virtually all of the commercially available lavender oil is derived from farm raised plants. What's more, there are dozens of varieties of the farm raised species, which are mere hybrids used primarily for perfumery and floral purposes. Bissas notes that these types are "less potent and...inferior to the true lavender." Oil of Lavender by North American Herb & Spice Co. is the "true" lavender, plus it is guaranteed 100% wild lavender harvested from the deep Mediterranean. In fact, it is the only guaranteed wild high mountain lavender available. The lavender utilized grows wild in the mountains as high as 6000 feet above sea level and is free of chemicals, pesticides, and/or solvents. This is the original wild lavender described by the ancients as a potent natural medicine. It is a most rare and precious oil. This wild lavender oil (in olive oil) makes a highly invigorating rub; apply it vigorously anywhere on the body. Use a few drops of this wild oil internally as needed.

Myrtle oil

The leaves of the myrtle bush, a native of the Mediterranean, are the source of a unique and versatile essential oil. The leaves and flowers, which are highly aromatic, have been used both in food and as medicine.

Myrtle has been used as a health aid for the skin and respiratory system for thousands of years. The ancient Greeks relied upon myrtle as a skin tonic for enhancing beauty and for healing damaged tissues. It was also used for curing bladder infections, wounds, and skin diseases.

Today, the primitives still administer myrtle for a wide range of conditions. In North Africa it is relied upon as an anti-diabetic agent. In Turkey it is used to reverse chronic cough and for alleviating sinus distress. The Turks also use it for diabetes. Modern research documents that myrtle truly is a fighter of diabetes, finding that it helps protect the pancreas from chemical induced damage. Hungarian researchers discovered that it also kills fungi, particularly the difficult to kill Candida albicans. Today, herbalists use myrtle for asthma, sinusitis, chronic cough, lung congestion, skin wounds, vaginitis, bladder infections, hemorrhoids, and sore throat. Rub it into the scalp to combat itching and dandruff.

Perhaps myrtle's greatest use is in the healing of skin. It is an invigorating tonic for normal skin as well as for aging skin. Yet, it is also invaluable for emergencies such as wounds, burns, abrasions, cuts, and scratches. It is specifically acknowledged for inducing the healing of damaged skin and mucous membranes. Apply it to virtually any skin wound or lesion. For instance, one women reported to me that the oil "eradicated" brown spots, which were due to sun damage, on her face.

Myrtle is also an exotic oil, that is it is an aphrodisiac. The smell alone is stimulating. Applied topically to the appropriate areas, it regenerates even the most feeble of sexual functions for both men and women.

N-acetyl cysteine (NAC)

This amino acid is currently available in emergency rooms for the treatment of drug overdose. It is particularly valuable for reversing poisoning by acetaminophen, the active ingredient of Tylenol.

The reversal of drug toxicity is the main use of NAC. In this respect it helps prevent and reverse drug induced liver damage and/or failure. However, it is also a proven aid for combating nuclear radiation. Thus, it is a versatile agent for aiding in the detoxification of harmful chemicals of all types.

Olive oil

A tin or two of olive oil would go a long way for aiding survival no matter what the disaster. Extra virgin olive oil is useful both as a nutrient rich food and a potent medicine. It is easily stored and has a prolonged shelf life. When opened, it rarely spoils.

Recently, an article illustrating the novel properties of olive oil was published in the reputable journal, *Nutrition Reviews*. The authors discovered that olive oil's beneficial effects go far beyond its vegetable/healthy fat content. The oil contains a variety of powerful antioxidants known as polyphenols. Apparently, it is these compounds which account for olive oil's therapeutic properties. While the researchers note that olive oil research is "in its infancy," the fact is this God-blessed substance has been relied upon as a survival food, as well as medicine, since the beginning of time.

Olive oil may be preserved virtually indefinitely by adding certain herbs/spices. After opening, crumple and add fresh wild sage, oregano, cumin, and/or rosemary. Or, even more conveniently, add oil of sage, oregano, cumin, and/or rosemary. Simply add 5 to 10 drops of these oils per quart of oil. This will prevent oxidation of the oil after it is opened. One study determined that the oil's shelf life was increased nine-fold by simply adding antioxidant spices/herbs.

Oregano

Anything powerful enough to destroy sewage but harmless to the human body would be of great value in difficult times. It was Jean Valnet, M. D., in *The Practice of Aromatherapy*, who described how a researcher named Cavel stumbled upon it. Cavel searched the plant kingdom for germ killing substances, deciding that essential oils were the most powerful. To evaluate them he used sewage water and fed it beef broth to stimulate growth. Various oils were added, one at a time, to determine antiseptic activity. Oil of oregano was among the most powerful, completely sterilizing the water in a 1% concentration. Other powerful antiseptics included oil of orange, lemongrass, cinnamon, and clove as well as lavender, cumin, and rosemary. It took nearly six times the amount of synthetic germicides to equal the power of wild oregano oil. In fact, all of the aforementioned antiseptic oils were more powerful than the synthetic. Incredibly, wild oregano oil was 6.5 times more effective than garlic oil, the latter being notoriously respected as one of the most powerful natural germ killers. Thyme was also exceptionally high, that is wild thyme (*Thymus vulgaris*). However, the latter is less commonly consumed as a food, so its internal use is less respected compared to highly edible substances such as oregano, cumin, rosemary, cinnamon, and lemongrass. Wild thyme from the edible species might be useful as a topical antiseptic, but it must be emulsified in olive oil. Note: wild thyme is entirely different than the commercially available *Thymus capitus,* which is unfit for human consumption.

Cavel's work is corroborated by modern research. In 1998 microbiologist Daniel Fung and colleagues at Kansas State University discovered that oregano impedes the growth of E. coli, preventing it from infecting the body. Siddiqui found (*Medical Science Research*, 1996) that oil of oregano was so powerful against viruses that it caused "disintegration", which was observed under the electron microscope. The respected Cornell University proved that oregano, even as a spice, killed all 30 organisms against which it was tested, including E. coli and Salmonella.

These modern findings merely edify the historical record. It was Fleisher who thoroughly documented the fact that wild oregano is Bible Hyssop. The ancient Hebrew text contains the word *ezov,* which was erroneously translated as "hyssop." Furthermore, Maimonides, the 12th century Jewish physician of Islamic Spain, made it evident that the hyssop of the Law is simply the wild oregano that grows in the mountains. Earl Smith, Bible researcher, notes that the burning bush of Moses is likely the wild oregano that grew on Mt. Sinai. This makes sense, since Moses unquestionably had to combat plague and pestilence during his prolonged and arduous tour, and, certainly, God's guidance is oriented for physical as well as spiritual benefits.

Oil of oregano is an edible oil made from wild mountain-grown oregano. To be edible the spice must be the *wild mountain oregano* found in the hot climate of the Mediterranean. European, Spanish, and/or so called Mexican oreganos have not been subjected to the rigorous research as have the deep Mediterranean types. What's more, true original oreganos are not found in Europe or Spain.

Mexican oregano isn't oregano. Rather, it is listed in botany books as an entirely different plant of the *Lippia* genus. It is rarely useful as a medicinal oregano and is also inferior as a spice.

Currently, there is a lack of continuity in the essential oil market. Plus, there is a deficiency of aggressive quality control. With regards to oregano oil Julia Lawless confirms this confusion in the *Encyclopedia of Essential Oils*, saying that the typical commercial oregano oil is not a true oregano but is either marjoram or Thymus. This is because the commercial oils have not been carefully screened to be sure they are edible. North American Herb & Spice originated the use of edible Oil of Oregano. This is the real wild 100% Mediterranean oregano and is free of non-oregano plants like Spanish thyme or Mexican Lippia. With the North American oil quality control is exceptional and raw material sourcing rigorous. The wild oregano is picked by hand high in the Mediterranean mountains. One ton of the raw spice produces a mere 8 kilograms of oil. It is extracted only with steam.

Beware of oils made from cheap imitations which are not edible and/or which are made from Spanish thyme (Thymus capitus), Origanum vulgare (i.e. marjoram), or Mexican sage. Do not consume these types internally.

Recently, there has developed a trend to genetically engineer virtually everything. Unfortunately, soon, spices, including oregano, will be genetically produced. Genetically engineered spices must be farm raised on commercially treated soils or in greenhouses. Furthermore, the seed is produced by cloning, in other words, it is genetically altered. The purveyors of these genetically reconstituted spices are aggressively attempting to market their wares. They hope to "standardize" oregano and other spices by growing them in the laboratory. Genetically engineered spices/herbs are inferior to the wild types. These are not the types of antiquity, the Hyssop of the Bible, the wild oregano of the Law. Only the substances growing in the Fertile Crescent are of the correct biblical species. Only wild oregano is the basis of modern research elucidating medicinal powers. North American did the research and supplies guaranteed wild oregano from the Fertile Crescent, hand picked in the mountains and valleys of the Mediterranean. Ask for wild oregano, because that is the highest in quality and safest for human consumption. Plus, the wild oregano is the type which has been utilized by societies since the beginning of human history and which is unaltered by human hands. Wild oil of oregano may be ordered by calling 1-800-243-5242, or check in finer health stores and pharmacies for the distinctive blue label with the white medicine dropper cap.

In summary, the properties of oil of oregano proven by modern research include:

• destruction of all molds and fungi
• disintegration of RNA and DNA viruses, including herpes viruses
• inhibition of bacterial growth, including staph, strep, and E. coli
• destruction of the parasite, *Giardia lamblia*
• destruction of mold spores in the air
• halting of the growth and/or destruction of skin fungi
• increasing the output of bile
• reversing pain and inflammation
• improving the detoxification capacities of the liver

Note that virtually all of the research has been done using wild oregano from the deep Mediterranean, not Spanish oregano, Spanish thyme, Thymus capitus, T. capitus, or thymol. The types that are consumable either as oil or herb are the edible oreganos from the Mediterranean and Middle East. These are similar to the types used in the spice trade but are of a higher quality and purity.

The point is simple: for internal consumption the spice must be edible, plus it should be the type upon which the majority of the significant research has been performed. It must be the type which has been utilized since antiquity and which is safe for internal consumption in any form.

There are three forms of wild oregano available: the oil, the crushed herb, and the juice. The oil is extracted from the high mountain spice, which grows up to 8000 feet above sea level. The juice is produced by a special process, which yields the water soluble fractions from the spice. It is a natural source of oxygenated compounds and flavonoids. The crushed herb is precisely the same spice known as Bible Hyssop, which grows on mineral rich mountain soil. In fact, this oregano often grows directly on rock. Thus, it is a dense source of naturally occurring minerals, particularly calcium, magnesium, phosphorus, iodine, and potassium. Known as Oregamax capsules, this is a village formula, consisting of wild oregano, Rhus coriaria (mountain sumac berry), garlic, and onion. Interestingly, all of the aforementioned spices are natural antiseptics. North American Herb & Spice's oil of oregano and Oregamax capsules are 100% wild and are *not* genetically engineered.

Pantothenic acid

This should be regarded as the "speed healing" vitamin. This is because this vitamin accelerates the healing of virtually any injury and is particularly reliable for aiding in the recovery from trauma. It accelerates the healing of a wide range of wounds/injuries, including post-surgical wounds, bed sores, broken bones, sprains, burns, stomach ulcers, and bruises.

Pantothenic acid, or vitamin B_5, is critical for the function of every internal organ. It plays a basic role in the metabolism of food and is also essential for the proper utilization of numerous other vitamins. It is required for the metabolism of protein, carbohydrate, and fatty acids, in other words, virtually every function within the body is dependent upon it. It is the key vitamin responsible for stimulating the synthesis of natural cortisone, which largely accounts for its wound healing actions. The vitamin also offers significant anti-stress powers. In fact, inability to cope with stress is one of the major symptoms of its deficiency. Top sources of naturally occurring pantothenic acid include royal jelly, organ meats, peanut butter, salmon, and eggs. It is notable that these foods are rarely consumed currently. Thus, pantothenic acid deficiency is endemic, that is the majority of Westerners suffer from the deficiency.

Red grape powder (Resvitanol™)

Like spices, grapes and grape extracts have been relied upon medicinally from the beginning of time. They are mentioned with a hint of medicinal value in all of the holy books, particularly the Qur'an. Such grapes of antiquity were obviously of a type different than commercial American grapes.

Due to its alcohol content wine is contraindicated during a crisis. Nor is it a reliable cure for disease. Fortunately, there are other ways to achieve the health benefits of grapes without drinking wine. This is because there are other means to concentrate the healing attributes of grapes. These powers are found primarily in a family of chemicals known as polyphenols (or merely phenols). Researchers at the University of Denmark determined that phenols found in the pure grape, notably the skin of red grapes, worked equally as well as wine in reversing circulatory damage and preventing cardiovascular disease. The researchers produced a concentrate from the grape skins, which are a residue of the wine industry. These grape skin/seed antioxidants are among the most potent agents for protecting the blood vessels and heart from toxic damage.

The medicinal properties of grapes are being heartily investigated by hundreds of researchers. Yet, the true power is found in the whole grape, the skin, seed, as well as the vine, and leaf. Red or purple grape extracts provide components which are highly protective against heart disease, cancer, and arthritis. A recent report published in the *Journal of Biological Chemistry* indicates that a grape compound, known as resveratrol, may be more effective than common drugs, such as aspirin, in reversing or preventing arthritis, heart disease, cancer, and even Alzheimer's disease. The compound completely blocked the toxic reaction which precipitates these diseases. What's more, researchers believe that this effect may explain why individuals living in regions where fresh grapes form a large part of the diet have a much reduced incidence of heart disease and cancer. The active ingredient of the grape extracts is a potent flavonoid called *resveratrol.*

Italian researchers discovered something even more profound regarding the chemistry of resveratrol. They determined that this unique chemical revitalizes nerve cells. In fact, resveratrol induced portions of the nerves to regenerate, in other words, the nerves started growing again, a feat formerly deemed impossible. A reasonable conclusion is that resveratrol is a major protector of the genes, in other words, it prevents chromosome damage. Yet, grape extracts offer another mechanism of action. Apparently, they are directly toxic to cancer cells. Researcher S. Joshi found that when grape seed extract was placed in the test tube with various cancer cells, some of the cells were killed. H. Preuss of Georgetown University also made this determination, finding that an extract of grape seed inhibited the growth of human cancers, killing some cancer cells outright, while increasing the strength of normal cells. Other researchers have determined that the red grape components offer significant anti-pain and anti-inflammation powers.

Imagine the benefits to the human body by naturally concentrating the medicinal components of grapes. Such a grape extract, as a natural antiinflammatory, anti-toxic, and anti-cancer agent, would have potentially lifesaving actions. It was Dr. Folts from the University of Wisconsin who proclaimed that a pill of *concentrated grape flavonoids,* not just one or two synthetic components, would be powerful preventive medicine for Americans. Fortunately, now such a product is available. Known as *Resvitanol* it is the only grape product available that provides all of the components from the grape without the sugar. A "village formula," it is made in a primitive fashion, which preserves its therapeutic essence. The entire red grape bunch is sun-ripened for a prolonged period. As a result, the sugar is extracted by the sun: the best remains: the minerals, flavonoids, and vitamins which are naturally concentrated in the vine, seed, skin, and leaves.

Resvitanol is made from pulverized wilderness red grapes.

Thus, it is a truly unprocessed grape product, the only such product available made from not only the seeds and skin but also the vine and leaves. Did you know that many of the commercial grape products are processed with solvents? With Resvitanol you get all of the benefits of the grape without the chemicals.

Resvitanol is a dense source of flavonoids, vitamins, and trace minerals. It is one of the most mineral packed and nutrient dense substances ever analyzed. The analysis revealed that it is an excellent source of a wide range of minerals, notably calcium, magnesium, chromium, potassium, iron, and silica. Incredibly, it contains some 1500 mg of potassium per 100 grams, making it far richer in this mineral than any fruit or vegetable. A superb source of chromium, it contains nearly 1400 mcg per 100 grams, which makes it incredibly dense in this mineral. Its natural chromium content is perhaps the most impressive component. A mere two teaspoons contains nearly 100% of the minimum daily need for this mineral, which makes it richer than virtually any other natural food product known. Natural calcium levels are high at 440 mg per 100 grams; compare this to whole milk at 120 mg per 100 grams. It is also an excellent source of naturally occurring vitamin C, containing some 150 mg per 100 grams (about 8 mg of crude natural vitamin C per teaspoon), making it far superior as a source of this nutrient to any fruit or vegetable, even orange juice. This high vitamin C content is to be expected from a truly mountain raised sun ripened substance. Thus, Resvitanol is a tremendously rich source of natural nutrients, and this is rare to find in herb/vitamin capsules. This is the original crude red grape food, completely sun-dried and totally natural. Resvitanol creates a new definition in what is a nutritional supplement.

The uniqueness of Resvitanol is related to the fact that the majority of nutrients in the grape are found not in the seed but in the skin, vine, and pulp. Thus, this formula provides not only the various flavonoids, such as the OPCs and resveratrol, but also an enormous density of nutrients.

There is yet another group of ingredients unique to red grape extract: organic acids such as tartaric and malic acids. According to Blumgarten theses substances are effective stimulants for the digestion and elimination as well as for the kidneys. This may be why grapes have long been utilized as a detoxification aid as well as kidney/digestive tonic.

Rosemary

Rosemary is a highly beneficial medicinal herb. Ignored by Americans as little more than a flavoring, it has an ancient history primarily as a medicine rather than a food.

The wisdom of the ancients regarding rosemary has been confirmed by modern research. Studies show that rosemary is among the most potent antioxidants known. This means that for survival purposes, it is infinitely more valuable than minor antioxidants such as vitamin E and beta carotene.

Rosemary is a potent antioxidant for all tissues. It possesses significant anti-cancer and anti-toxic powers. However, it's antioxidant actions are geared more directly for the brain and other tissues of the nervous system, which depend upon fat soluble antioxidants. Rosemary is one of the most readily absorbed of all fat soluble antioxidants and efficiently finds its way into nerve tissues. It is rapidly absorbed via inhalation, through the skin, and via the digestive tract.

The easiest way to get the amount of rosemary needed to achieve these effects is via supplements, either herbal capsules or edible rosemary oil. Don't use rosemary extracts, that is standardized products. Duke notes that studies show whole plant supplements are more effective than single components or "standardized" chemicals in anti-toxic action.

Rosemary is listed among the most ancient of all medicinal herbs. For thousands of years it has been known particularly for its ability to improve the function of the mind. Ancient texts describe how concoctions of rosemary were used to stimulate the mind, enhance mood, boost intellectual powers, and improve memory. In fact, it is most famous as a memory aid. Yet, it was also famous for combating disorders of the nerves as well as arthritis. Oil of rosemary is a concentrate of this herb's healing capacities. Condensed power is ultra-important in any crisis, including chronic disease.

Modern research documents how rosemary works. Researchers describe it as having unusually high antioxidant activity, far greater than mere vitamins. Other researchers note that oil of rosemary is a strong inhibitor of viruses. Dr. Navarro found that the oil is highly protective for the liver, especially when it is damaged by toxic chemicals. French doctors found that oil of rosemary actually doubled the output of bile, which helps purge the liver of toxins. Furthermore, this function of stimulating the flow of bile is helpful in human nutrition, because this substance is direly needed for the digestion of fat. In the Middle East rosemary is used currently for digestive problems, but not just for the liver: it is applied for spastic colon, excess gas, heartburn, and indigestion. Europeans use rosemary as a circulatory stimulant. Chevalier describes its value in improving circulation, especially for the brain. Virtually all illnesses are associated with poor circulation. Topically, it is a great stimulant to the scalp, improving blood flow. Rosemary has an ancient history for fighting pain. It is still used for this purpose in Europe. Michael Tierra, master herbalist, notes that rosemary is of "great benefit in treating headaches," because it contains natural anti-pain compounds.

Rosemary is also an incredibly powerful anti-mutagenic substance. This means it combats virtually any toxic chemical which damages the genes. Thus, rosemary is of lifesaving importance in the event of toxic chemical exposure. Researchers in England found that rosemary extract thoroughly protected the genetic material from chemical induced damage, partly by stimulating the synthesis of anti-toxic enzymes such as glutathione. The researchers concluded that rosemary can increase the body's ability to dispose of noxious chemicals. Few natural substances offer this power. In fact, of over 140 fruits, herbs, and spices tested, rosemary was one of the rare few that proved to be a gene protector. The point is you must have this substance available in order to achieve guaranteed protection against toxic chemical exposures, radiation poisoning, as well as the stresses of everyday life in the modern world. The individual who wishes to be assured of protection against the poisonous future must have rosemary available, as oil of rosemary, wild rosemary capsules, as well as the bulk herb. The rat study by Dr. Milner at Penn State tells all: rats who were fed rosemary were twice as likely to escape being damaged by toxic chemicals than those who ate no rosemary.

Royal jelly

This is the food utilized by what is perhaps the most important creature on the earth: the queen bee. Royal jelly is super-rich in vitamins, minerals, and enzymes. Plus, it contains the bonus of naturally occurring steroids, which are of enormous utility for the function of the human body.

Few people realize how critical royal jelly is; it is the only substance making the difference between the long lived queen bee and regular bees. Incredibly, the queen lives 24 times as long as the regular bees, plus she is stronger and sexually potent. This explains why royal jelly is famous for halting impotence and improving hormone balance. It also explains its ancient use for rejuvenation, for healthier skin, and for halting aging. It is perhaps the most ancient of all beauty aids.

Modern research shows royal jelly has powerful effects upon adrenal function, and, thus, helps combat stress. This is largely because it is the richest source of a critical vitamin, pantothenic acid, which is essential for the proper function of these glands. Plus, it is high in naturally occurring steroids, that is cortisone-like substances. Adrenal weakness is due to cortisone deficiency. Symptoms of weak adrenals include exhaustion (which doesn't improve with sleep), nervousness, menstrual difficulties, depression or anxiety, digestive disturbances, chronic headaches, allergies, inability to handle stress, chronic upper back pain, sweaty palms, cold extremities, and cravings for salt and/or sugar. In Europe royal jelly is famous for reversing adrenal failure as well as female sexual or menstrual disorders. For fighting fatigue, nervousness, or panic attacks royal jelly is essential. Natural pantothenic acid is rare in most foods; the only common sources are liver and eggs; few Americans eat these. Thus, royal jelly offers hundreds of natural substances, just as God made them, plus the rare natural pantothenic acid, which is much more powerful and useful than the synthetic. The consumption of royal jelly is an excellent means to achieve a daily intake of crude unprocessed pantothenic acid. Use nature's special remedies and gain ideal health, *just like the queen.*

Royal jelly is available in three forms: the lypholized powder, that is the dry capsule, the fresh liquid, which must be frozen or refrigerated, and the newly available stabilized liquid. The latter, which is a convenient means of consuming fresh royal jelly, is available as Royal Oil. This type can be conveniently consumed under the tongue for optimal effect. For capsules the pantothenic acid-fortified Royal Kick is available. It contains a guaranteed potency of the active ingredient, 10-hydroxydecanoic acid (10-HDA).

Note: natural source steroids, such as those found in royal jelly, are harmless. These beneficial substances have been used for centuries.

Sage

An ancient proverb claims that if sage is consumed every day, the individual shall never grow old. During Medieval times the English insisted that this herb was necessary for good health. These ancient findings are supported by modern research. Sage is one of the most powerful herbal antioxidants known. Researchers determined that when sage is added to food, the shelf life is extended tremendously—even longer than with synthetic preservatives. Could this same action occur within humans?

With the plethora of information disseminated about the protective effects of natural antioxidants, such as vitamin E, vitamin C, and Pycnogenol™, it is revealing that an edible herb like sage is significantly more powerful. According to Taintu sage superceded virtually every substance tested in halting oxidation of fats. Edible sage oil from the wild spice is the type useful for human health. Sage oil is potent. Only small amounts are necessary, like 3 to 10 drops daily. Larger amounts may be needed to combat toxic chemical exposure. It can be freely used topically on wounds, cuts, abrasions, skin irritations, burns, warts, etc. It makes an excellent gargle for sore throats and can be applied to canker sores and cold sores as often as needed. Do not consume commercial or aromatherapy (i.e. clary) sage oils internally.

Sage is also a digestive tonic. It is particularly valuable for inflammation in the intestines, that is colitis and irritable bowel. Plus, it is soothing to the nerves of the digestive tract. Historically, herbalists have relied upon sage for diarrhea as well as intestinal parasites.

If the nervous system is out of balance, sage is perhaps the ideal tonic. It exerts tremendous calming action upon the nerves. Herbalists currently rely upon it for anxiety, nervousness, agitation. They even massage it into the skin to relieve muscle tension and pain. Furthermore, it is used for reversing depression and apathy, because of its ability to boost mood and stimulate the mind. Sage is an invaluable mind activator.

Sage is especially valuable as a hormone tonic. It gives great strength to the adrenal glands, which are responsible for controlling energy, the ability to fight stress, and the resistance to disease. In the modern era everyone needs an adrenal tonic. Sage also exerts powerful effects upon the sex hormone system. A partial list of conditions for which sage oil has been reported helpful includes:

- cold hands/feet or low body temperature
- immune decline
- sore throat/laryngitis
- fatigue and weakness
- adrenal weakness (and to combat high stress)
- respiratory conditions, particularly asthma
  and whooping cough
- insomnia
- hot flashes
- imbalances in menstruation/PMS
- infertility and impotence
- prostate disorders
- reducing of excessive sweating
- depression/anxiety
- agitation
- irregular menses
- hair loss
- dandruff

- aging skin
- graying of the hair
- muscular tension

What's more, sage is a beauty aid. Since ancient times it has been taken to reverse graying of the hair. Use it as a scalp/hair conditioner. Add it to facial tonics to greatly improve the tone/beauty of the skin. Sage is an astringent when applied to the skin, meaning it is a drying agent, counteracting excessive oiliness, scaling, and perspiration. However, since edible Oil of Sage is emulsified in extra virgin olive oil, it can be used on scaly and/or dry skin. For excessive graying, use internally as well as externally. Note: Sage oil should not be consumed by breast feeding mothers, since it tends to slow milk production. DO NOT use commercial or aromatherapy sage oil. It may be high in adulterants and/or thujone, which is potentially toxic. Don't use sage oil if pregnant or nursing. Even so, remember, sage is an edible spice. Edible sage is the type consumed daily in the Mediterranean as a tea and tonic. Inherently, as a natural mountain spice it is safe for human consumption.

St. John's Wort

This is one of the most reliable anti-stress and nerve protective substances known. Since ancient times, St. John's wort has been utilized to combat mood imbalances, mental stress, and depression. Yet, it was also regarded as sort of miracle cure for various wounds, including internal ulcers, skin wounds, burns, and cuts.

St. John's wort contains a wide array of unique compounds. It is an excellent source of flavonoids, which is made obvious by the fact that it consists largely of brightly colored yellow or yellow-orange flowers. According to the latest research the flavonoids, notably a compound known as *hyperforin*, appear to be the major active ingredients accounting for its brain enhancing, wound healing, and anti-stress actions. Chemically, these flavonoids act by helping the brain produce neurotransmitters such as serotonin, noradrenalin, and dopamine. The latter is required for blocking the ill effects of Parkinson's disease as well as Alzheimer's. In other words, St. John's wort contains chemicals which protect the brain from aging.

Crude St. John's wort contains a variety of natural compounds with potent biological activity. Wild-growing St. John's wort is much higher in active ingredients than farm raised. The wild herb is rich in compounds known as *dianthrones*, which are relatively rare chemicals. Hypericin, St. John's wort's most highly touted active ingredient, is a dianthrone. The herb is also a good source of carotenoids, including certain types that combat toxic chemical exposure and cancer. What's more, recently it was discovered that St. John's wort is one of the few plants which contains a considerable amount of naturally occurring melatonin. This combined with the fact that it contains the calming neurotransmitter GABA (gamma amino butyric acid) largely explains its brain enhancing/antidepressive properties. It is also high in essential oil, which has been a favorite remedy of herbalists for hundreds of years. The essential oil was famous in Medieval times for its wound healing properties.

Unprocessed St. John's wort that is rich in flavonoids is a reliable natural remedy for defeating the mental stress associated with failure to cope or severe psychic pressure. It is also a dependable cure for apathy, grief, and depression. The key to achieving significant results is to select a St. John's wort product high in naturally occurring flavonoids. It was previously believed that a specific chemical, called hypericin, was the major component responsible for curative effects. However, Laakmann and Schellenberg, publishing in Germany, have thoroughly determined that it is the flavonoids that are mostly responsible for this herb's therapeutic powers. Essentially, if the product is low in flavonoids, it fails to work. This makes sense, since a plethora of research points to the critical role of flavonoids as the medicinal ingredients of plants.

Look for St. John's wort products which contain naturally occurring flavonoids, not just hypericin. The label may not supply this information, because this data is so new. Unprocessed St. John's wort from wild plants is superior to farm raised. Be sure that the supplier certifies that the product is made from the flowering tops rather than the lower stems. If possible, request an assay from the manufacturer describing flavonoid content.

Where this plant grows has a great impact upon its therapeutic powers. St. John's wort is a native of North Africa, Eastern Europe, and the Mediterranean. Thus, plants from these regions are top grade. In summary, the primary therapeutic powers of St. John's wort are as follows:

- for combating depression
- for balancing mood
- for aiding in the healing of wounds (either the oil or pure herb)
- as an anti-viral agent, particularly against herpes
- for relieving stress and improving stress tolerance
- for relieving head pain, particularly migraine/cluster headaches (the high flavonoid type only)

Note: for a guaranteed wild mountain-grown Mediterranean—and high flavonoid—St. John's wort, see Appendix A.

Salt

Salt saves lives, especially in harsh circumstances. It has always saved lives. It has never been a killer. However, the medical profession caused it to appear as the enemy. Now medical scientists are withdrawing their salt warnings. The fact is they have admitted that aggressively removing salt from the diet is dangerous. Researchers publishing in 1998 in the prestigious British journal, the *Lancet,* found that the regular intake of salt had a slightly protective effect in preserving life and preventing sudden death. Dr. Alderman of New York's Albert Einstein Hospital provided definitive proof. He began studying the value of salt in heart patients after discovering accidentally that heart patients who died suddenly had low salt levels. By giving salt to heart patients premature deaths were essentially halted, and the survival rate improved by some 400%. In other words, individuals with the lowest levels of salt in their bodies were most likely to die.

In ancient times salt was traded as a valuable commodity, and in some regions it was equal in value to its weight in gold. There were specific health reasons it was so highly esteemed. Now we are rediscovering that our bodies require salt, and, if we become seriously deficient in this nutrient, our lives are at risk.

Salt, as sodium chloride, is the most important electrolyte of the blood. In fact, 90% of the mineral content of the blood consists of it. This is why blood tastes salty. Salt is rapidly depleted from the body during periods of stress. It must be replaced or the health will suffer. Both extremely hot and cold weather cause salt depletion.

Certain individuals suffer from a condition which I've named the *Salt Wasting Syndrome*. I first discovered this dangerous condition in my clinic in Arlington Heights, Illinois. Some symptoms of this condition were identified and enumerated, but no one had previously recognized that it occurs within so many individuals. As many as 20 million Americans suffer from it. The condition is the result of the inability of the body to produce adequate amounts of adrenal steroids, specifically the salt retaining hormone known as *aldosterone*. Thus, despite a normal or even above normal intake of salt, the individual loses it essentially faster than it is consumed. This may be represented by a low or low normal sodium and/or chloride level in the blood. This largely explains why certain individuals ravenously crave salt. It is a protective mechanism within their bodies that is in action. In the extreme salt deficiency can be serious, leading to vascular collapse and shock, perhaps death. Sodium is required for maintaining blood flow and pressure. Symptoms of salt deficiency include:

- exhaustion
- spastic muscles
- leg/foot cramps
- poor appetite
- headaches
- paranoia and/or psychotic behavior
- nausea
- confusion and/or irritability
- dizziness
- cold extremities
- sluggish circulation
- anxiety and depression
- impaired memory

Salt is a strength providing nutrient. Plus, it is a preservative. What's more, it is an invaluable aid in combating stress due its positive actions on the adrenal glands. It must be available as part of the everyday combat kit. Sea salt is the finest type to consume. Procure the highest quality sea salt available. Ideally, opt for salt which has undergone the least amount of processing, i. e. crude unbleached sea or land salt. Remember, all land salt was once sea salt.

Selenium

Selenium is perhaps the most important of all protective trace minerals. It is an exceptionally powerful activator of cellular defenses. It offers enormous utility for cellular function by keeping critical cells, such as white blood, spleen, and liver cells, in a heightened state of alert. It is particularly valuable for combating toxic chemical and heavy metal poisoning.

Selenium offers dependable anti-cancer actions. Some 100 studies point to its indisputable role in cancer prevention. A recent study by *JAMA* showed that simply taking this mineral in a dose of 200 mcg daily cut in half the risk for lung, colon, and prostate cancers. That is an incredibly powerful response for a single substance, making it perhaps the most protective mineral/nutrient against cancer. Besides prevention selenium may help destroy cancer after it develops. One study found that taking selenium dramatically improved survival in individuals with colon and/or rectal cancer. These results indicate that selenium enhances the body's ability to ward off damage due to poisons of all types. This is largely due to the fact that it is required for the production of an enzyme that protects every cell and organ in the body from any insult: glutathione peroxidase. Researchers have shown that all living creatures have one element in common: they produce glutathione peroxidase. The enzyme is the initial defense for all animals from insects to humans against harmful stressors, including toxic chemicals, radiation, UV light, and free radicals.

Selenium is required for the cellular response against poisonous compounds. Without it, cells are readily destroyed. A lack of selenium increases the potency of toxic chemicals.

Researchers found that in the absence of this mineral the liver is readily damaged by synthetic chemicals, and when selenium is given the damage is minimized, even reversed. Their conclusion is that selenium protects the chromosomes from being damaged by toxic chemicals. Therefore, when glutathione levels are diminished, the tissues are easily traumatized. Selenium is responsible for regulating glutathione production, and, thus, a lack of it leaves the body highly vulnerable to toxic chemical induced damage.

To boost glutathione synthesis take supplemental vitamin E, selenium, riboflavin, and vitamin C. These are the most important glutathione increasing vitamins. Herbs/spices that boost glutathione levels include cumin, oregano, rosemary, and sage. Other herbs are helpful, but the aforementioned are the most aggressive and powerful. For instance, one study found that cumin oil alone increased tissue glutathione levels by nearly 700%, while rosemary boosted levels by some 400%. Taking the vitamins along with the herbs/spices dramatically improves the operations of the internal glutathione factories, giving the individual ideal health as well as the best chances for surviving a toxic crisis.

Supplemental selenium and selenium-rich foods, such as Brazil nuts and garlic, may provide lifesaving protection in the event of a chemical exposure, radiation contamination, or sudden illness. If you are exposed to poisonous chemicals and/or radioactivity, take selenium immediately, at least 400 mcg twice daily. Be sure to consume only organically bound types, that is selenium chelates and/or selenium kelp.

Recently, an excellent type of organically bound selenium has become available. Researched at Rutgers University *selenium cruciferate* is a highly absorbable sulfur/amino acid-bound selenium. It is the type of selenium naturally found in high selenium vegetables like mustard greens, cabbage, broccoli, and kale. The selenium is in the form of selenomethionine and selenocysteine, which are the ideal types to consume. Selenium cruciferate is an exceptionally high grade nutritional supplement.

Large amounts of selenium are for short term consumption only, like two or three weeks. The normal daily dosage is 200 to 600 mcg, depending upon the individual chemistry and/or level of exposure to toxins. Also, eat selenium rich foods such as Brazil nuts, onions, and garlic. Yet, the point is in the event of a massive toxic chemical or radiation release, high amounts, like 1000 mg or more, of organically bound selenium taken daily on a short term basis would be lifesaving.

Tomatoes

The tomato's greatest attribute isn't its vitamins. It is a compound known as lycopene, the component which gives tomatoes their brilliant red color. Researchers have determined that this pigment, which is chemically related to beta carotene, is as much as 10 times more powerful than beta carotene as an antioxidant. It is one of nature's most effective cancer fighters. Plus, it is a stimulant to the function of virtually every cell in the body. This is because lycopene aids in the transport of oxygen, which is the fuel that drives cellular metabolism.

Lycopene exerts strong protective effects against cancer, but it also protects against toxic chemical exposure. Researchers determined that when cells are placed under severe stress lycopene prevents their degeneration. Apparently, lycopene improves the ability of cells to communicate with each other, helping them block the formation of tumor cells. In other words, it helps cells remain in their normal configuration, preventing them from degenerating into malignant cells.

Lycopene is found in only a few foods, notably red sweet peppers, red grapefruit, watermelon, apricots, papayas, and tomatoes, the latter being the richest source. However, these foods eaten alone are not a reliable source of therapeutic amounts. This is because lycopene is fat soluble, meaning it must be dissolved in fat to be taken into the blood. To gain optimal lycopene power eat concentrated sources of tomatoes. Tomato juice is a good source, but it must be mixed with a bit of extra virgin olive oil. Plain sun dried tomatoes or, preferably, sun dried tomatoes in olive oil provide a huge supply of lycopene. Tomato paste is another option, but be sure to mix it in a bit of extra virgin olive oil before consuming. If you are exposed to toxic chemicals, eat a can of tomato paste blended with two tablespoons of olive oil per day. This tomato paste cocktail is perhaps the most convenient and powerful of all lycopene "supplements". It is preferable to get lycopene via food versus supplements, especially foods like cooked tomato sauce, which combine a source of natural oil with the lycopene.

Vitamin A

Vitamin A is an important anti-stress agent. It strengthens immunity and boosts adrenal steroid synthesis. It is required for the formation of antibodies, which are essential for warding off infection. The antibodies protect the mucous membranes throughout the body from being attacked by pathogens. They are also needed to prevent allergic reactions.

Recently, researchers discovered that the regular intake of vitamin A impedes the growth of noxious viruses, particularly the herpes virus. In fact, a high vulnerability to herpes virus infection may warn of vitamin A deficiency. Researchers infected human cells with the virus. When the cells were "fed" vitamin A, the growth of the virus was dramatically reduced. The fact is vitamin A is the most powerful anti-viral vitamin known. Early in this century researchers discovered that if the body was deprived of vitamin A , all cells and organs degenerated. Animals fed vitamin A deficient diets became so frail that they looked as if they were starvation victims compared to the normally fed animals. Thus, during early research on this vitamin it became famous as the "growth factor." Indeed, now it is known that the growth of every cell in the human body is dependent upon it.

Vitamin C

In the early 1900s Dr. Szent-Gyorgi, a Hungarian biochemist, discovered that a crude extract from the adrenal glands of animals cured a variety of disorders. He also produced a similar curative extract from paprika. Later, he discovered that vitamin C was the major active ingredient in these foods, or at least he thought so. When Dr. Szent-Gyorgi purified the vitamin, it failed to produce the same curative effects. He concluded that crude extracts contain other components besides ascorbic acid accounting for the therapeutic properties. These substances were later named bioflavonoids.

Vitamin C and bioflavonoids are reliable, inexpensive remedies. Their uses are extensive, and they are among the easiest to take of all nutrients for combating toxic chemical exposure. They are universal toxin fighters, capable of reversing poisoning from virtually any compound. They reliably strengthen immunity. Plus, they exert anti-stress powers, largely due to their ability to increase adrenal steroid synthesis.

Incredibly, vitamin C deficiency may be more common today than it was early in this century. According to a recent study in the *Journal of the American College of Nutrition* millions of Americans are deficient in this life-saving vitamin. Random tests proved some 35% of individuals are lacking even the minimum requirement and up to 7% are severely deficient. The deficiencies were determined via blood testing. The point is in order for deficiencies to develop in the blood the individual must have been severely deficient. The fact is a large percentage of these individuals had signs/symptoms of borderline scurvy. What is perhaps most disturbing about these findings is the fact that this is occurring even though nearly half of all Americans take synthetic vitamin C in multiple vitamins or other supplements. The conclusion is the synthetic vitamin is poorly utilized and/or metabolized. It may be that the synthetic C is rejected by the cells as compared to the natural type and/or that it is not retained within the cells properly. Obviously, only natural vitamin C from food or food extracts offers reliable, prolonged—and 100% safe— protection.

Don't depend exclusively upon synthetic vitamin C in a life-threatening crisis. Rely instead on the immense powers of crude natural vitamin C plus the various flavonoids, the type only nature can produce. The vitamin C/flavonoid combination provides the individual with a type of condensed food, offering all of the unique benefits that only nature can provide. What's more, historically, only crude vitamin C sources have been applied to cure scurvy. Lemons and limes were used to reverse this disease in British sailors (17th century), pine needles cured it for Jacques Cartier and his men (16th century), and wild strawberry leaves salvaged George Washington and his army in Valley Forge. The natural ascorbic acid sources are the only time tested remedies.

Early symptoms of vitamin C deficiency are subtle and are rarely correctly surmised. Who would recognize fatigue, joint pain, joint stiffness, increased vulnerability to infections, slow recovery from illness, heat intolerance, and intolerance to exercise as early warning signs? A partial list of the symptoms of vitamin C deficiency include:

- severe fatigue
- irritability
- depression
- easy bruising/fragile blood vessels
- petechiae
- swollen, bleeding gums
- frequent colds/flu
- increased vulnerability to respiratory infections
- poor wound healing

Vitamin C is absolutely crucial for lung function. The vitamin improves the breathing capacity of the lungs and aids in the destruction of any germs that may enter them. What's more, it is of immense value for detoxification of the lungs in the event of noxious smoke or chemical inhalation. Vitamin C is rapidly destroyed by smoke. If it is replaced quickly, damage from smoke can be minimized, perhaps eliminated. The fact is researchers at Cornell University found that vitamin C was among the antioxidants which dramatically improved lung function, reducing the risk of—perhaps preventing—lung diseases such as asthma and emphysema.

Vitamin C's role in stress prevention is immense. It fights the toxic effects of stress upon both the immune and hormone systems. Dr. M. Levine, publishing in the *New England Journal of Medicine*, found that key immune cells do everything possible to concentrate vitamin C. The high level of the vitamin in these cells is apparently necessary so they can combat germs and kill cancer cells. Levine then discovered that immune cells ingest even more vitamin C when they are exposed to stress, which proves that the greater is the stress, the more is the need for the vitamin. Plus, whenever the body is exposed to stress, cold weather, hot weather, or toxic chemicals, vitamin C is dumped through the urine.

Natural source vitamin C exerts superior effects upon human tissues compared to the synthetic, plus it delivers a greater degree of biological activity. Note that virtually all of the significant research performed edifying the preventive role of vitamin C in human disease has been done with food, which clearly demonstrates the omnipotent role of natural vitamin C in the healing process. Thus, for optimal results don't rely on high dosages of synthetic vitamin C, like 5 to 10 grams daily, but instead depend upon high quality crude sources of ascorbic acid and the associated bioflavonoids. Or, use a combination of the synthetic plus the natural. Incredibly, a study done decades ago confirmed the unusual powers of natural vitamin C. The researchers found that vitamin C from natural sources was more powerful in its action than the synthetic type.

It is evident that the crude unprocessed ascorbic acid combined with with bioflavonoids is far more dependable for maximizing vitamin C's benefits. Bland writes in *Delicious Magazine* (1992) that vitamin C is always associated with bioflavonoids in nature and that at one time the latter were deemed so essential that they were named like a vitamin, i. e. *vitamin P*. He also notes that the flavonoids increase vitamin C's immune enhancing powers. This makes sense, because bioflavonoids exert a wide range of crucial functions. They maintain strong blood vessels; without them, the blood vessels degenerate. They may well be the crucial factor for preventing hardening of the arteries. The critical vitamin-like nature of these compounds is emphasized by original books on nutrition, such as Cooper's *Nutrition in Health and Disease*, which states that the bioflavonoids are necessary for the normal strength of the blood vessels.

Bioflavonoids are extremely potent antioxidants, far more powerful than vitamin C alone. What a mistake it is to isolate vitamin C, uncoupling it from its functional associates to which in nature it is so intimately bound. Flavonoids should stay combined with the vitamin C for optimal benefits. In a crisis depend upon crude ascorbate sources mixed with associated bioflavonoids. This type of agent will provide optimal results. Flavin-C is the highest state of this technology available, combining top grades of flavonoids with their associated vitamin C molecules. This is a balanced formula and is far more therapeutic than the synthetically derived alternatives. Flavin-C undergoes no adulterations and is free of synthetic vitamin C. It is guaranteed to be a true crude vitamin C/flavonoid source, like the type first discovered by Dr. Szent Gyorgi. Its ingredients include rose hip and acerola powder, immature orange powder, immature tangerine powder, immature grapefruit powder, and red grape powder, all of which are the top natural sources of vitamin C and bioflavonoids. Flavin-C is available in regular and non-citrus formulas in health stores, or to order direct call 1-800-243-5242. To order via the world wide web use the web site **www.wildspice.com**.

Vitamin D

Deficiency of this vitamin in Americans has reached epidemic proportions. As described by M. Thomas and colleagues in the *New England Journal of Medicine* as many as 40% of Americans are deficient, and this is despite the fact that many of these individuals are taking a daily multiple vitamin.

Vitamin D may not be a vitamin. It behaves within the cells like a hormone. The error in its definition makes sense. A vitamin is a substance that must be procured via the diet, in other words, it can't be produced in the body. Vitamin D fails to meet this definition, because if sunshine is available, the human body makes virtually all it needs.

Vitamin D is required for strong bones. It is needed to keep the teeth healthy and to prevent cavities. It is an impressive cancer blocker. It helps regulate cell growth. A regular supply is crucial for the maintenance of optimal health.

There are only two ways to get vitamin D: a well designed diet or, preferably, a combination of dietary sources plus exposure to sunshine. Only animal foods supply the vitamin. Top sources include eggs, butter, whole milk products, and fatty fish. Dark skinned people require a more prolonged exposure to the sun than light skinned individuals to achieve the same level of vitamin D synthesis. Individuals on strict diets and/or vegetarians are usually deficient. There is a warning: excessive sun exposure damages the skin, thus disrupting its ability to synthesize vitamin D. A few hours of indirect exposure, such as would occur from a long walk outdoors, is sufficient to procure daily vitamin D needs. Also, get your sun exposure before or after high noon. In fact, its a good idea to stay out of the sun during the summer months from 11:00 a.m. to 3:00 p.m. However, if exposure to the sun during this period is unavoidable, be sure to wear a wide brimmed hat.

Vitamin E

Vitamin E is useful for dozens of situations. In emergencies it is a versatile aid for the healing of virtually any wound, especially burns, cuts, and abrasions. It is particularly valuable for the healing of sunburns. Taken internally, it boosts the body's solar radiation defenses. What's more, it strengthens the immune system and improves the lungs' ability to detoxify poisonous compounds. Vitamin E is also a potent circulatory tonic and should be taken regularly by anyone with a history of heart disease.

The best vitamin E to use as an antioxidant is the crude unprocessed type. There are two categories: the mixed tocopherols and the tocotrienols. The tocopherol type is the most well known; it is usually made from soybean oil. The tocotrienol type is made from palm oil. Both serve as excellent antioxidants. However, recent research indicates that the newer type, the tocotrienols, may be superior as antioxidants for protecting the body against poisonous chemicals than the tocopherols. However, either type offers the actions sufficient for the recommendations of this book, because both are crude unprocessed natural extracts. Ideally, consume both types. Natural sources of tocotrienols include palm kernel oil, rice bran, rice germ, and nuts/seeds. Nutri-Sense is an excellent source of many of these food sources.

The antioxidant powers of vitamin E (or, more correctly, the *vitamins* E) are particularly valuable for protecting the skin and the lungs. Use it whenever these tissues are assaulted. Research points to the fact that the vitamin helps prevent scarring in the tissues when they are injured. Vitamin E has also recently been proven to offer valuable anti-aging properties for protecting the eyes. Individuals who regularly take the vitamin are much less likely to develop cataracts than those who fail to supplement. Even a small amount, like 400 I.U. every other day, was protective. Vitamin E's eye protecting powers would be greatly accelerated through the consumption of herb and spice antioxidants, particularly oil of rosemary, oil of oregano, oil of cumin, and oil of sage. Many of these oils contain crude natural vitamin E:

Case history: Mrs. P., a 75 year-old woman, went to her doctor because of failing vision. She was diagnosed with a cataract. A few months afterward she heard a radio program about the benefits of oil of oregano. She procured the product via mail (North American Herb & Spice Co.) and began regular consumption. Upon returning to her doctor, her eyes were examined by the head nurse. The nurse was shocked; Mrs. P.'s vision was normal and the cataract gone. The doctor rushed in and confirmed the exam and, like Mrs. P., gave the credit to her new-found remedy, oil of oregano, as well as Oregamax, which contains a variety of natural antioxidants, including gamma-tocopherol, the most biologically active form of vitamin E.

Vitamin E works synergistically with selenium. For optimal cataract protection take on a daily basis vitamin E, about 400 to 800 I.U. daily, 400 mcg of selenium, and herbal antioxidants such as oil of oregano and oil of rosemary, about 5 drops of each daily.

Zinc

Zinc has hit the news recently, because of the notorious zinc lozenges. The lozenges have been touted as a cure for colds. While they are not a cure, zinc is an important nutrient necessary for proper immune function. In this respect a regular intake helps strengthen immunity. This is because it is needed for fending off attacks by all types of germs. This explains why researchers, publishing in *Current Therapeutic Research*, discovered that zinc, as zinc acetate tablets, significantly reduced allergy and cold symptoms. The mineral is required for the synthesis of thymic hormones, which regulate immunity. What's more, zinc boosts the germ-killing capacity of white blood cells, plus it aids in the reproduction of these cells.

Perhaps zinc's greatest value relates to its role in wound healing. It is required for the synthesis and repair of all protein-based tissues, and that means skin, bone, muscles, and all other tissues in the human body. Zinc is also required for the daily healing of tissues from the damage that typically occurs as a result of aging and stress. This mineral is so critical that, without it, cellular repair and regeneration essentially halt. In fact, open wounds which fail to heal properly may signal a zinc deficiency. If an injury occurs, take zinc. A reasonable amount is 75 to 100 mg of a chelated zinc product taken daily until the wound/injury heals. Thereafter, take 25 to 50 mg daily. However, in the event of exposure to heavy metals, radiation, or poisonous gases, take more, such as 150 mg daily for several days. Such a high content of zinc can only be consumed for a short period of time, about a week or two. The reason is that high amounts of zinc interfere with copper metabolism, causing a copper deficiency. This ill effect is easily neutralized by taking copper on a daily basis, about 4 mg. Maintenance doses of zinc of 25 to 50 mg daily are safe and do not deplete copper reservoirs.

This antagonistic action of zinc with other metals has its value: it is a heavy metal antidote. Zinc aggressively competes with a variety of metals for absorption. Perhaps this is because it is so crucial for cellular function. In other words, the cells aggressively bind it. It is highly specific for blocking the absorption of cadmium, a heavy metal which causes lung and prostate disorders as well as cancer. Zinc also blocks the absorption of lead and other heavy metals. Whether exposed to heavy metals, toxic chemicals, smoke, radiation, or toxic gases, the consumption of zinc is a necessity.

Zinc is also a major nutrient for prostate health. Crude pumpkinseed oil is an excellent natural source of zinc. A special type of pumpkinseed oil is now available that is made from a unique variety of pumpkin, which grows in the pristine Steirermark region of southcentral Austria.

The history of this oil is fascinating. In 1773 the Austrian government deemed it so valuable that a directive was issued to protect it. The directive stated that it should be used only in salves, creams, and other medicinal products. Thus, it has been used as a natural medicine for hundreds of years.

This oil is concentrated, which makes it exceptionally nutrient dense. A mere quart of this extra virgin cold pressed oil requires the seeds of 33 pumpkins to produce. The oil's deep dark green color illustrates its tremendous content of chlorophyll, beta carotene, and vitamin E.

Austrian pumpkinseed oil is perhaps the best source of dietary zinc. A mere tablespoon, or one serving, contains a whopping 117 mg of zinc, which is an incredibly large amount. This is nearly 10 times the minimum requirement. This type of zinc is naturally bound and can be consumed in large amounts safely. A reasonable daily intake is from one to three tablespoons. As a natural zinc supplement consume a tablespoon or more on a daily basis.

Austrian pumpkinseed oil is a culinary delight. Drizzle it on salads, rice, whole grain pasta, and steamed vegetables. Add it to tomato juice, soups, and stir fry dishes (just before serving). This is an easy way to get your zinc and other vital nutrients in a healthy, tasty, and natural way.

High grade Austrian pumpkinseed oil may be difficult to find. For more information or to order call 1-800-243-5242.

CHAPTER 3

Nutrient Dense Foods

Food is critical to human survival. It must be carefully selected as a source of nutrients in order to maintain optimal health. The secret to procuring the greatest value from food is that it must be chosen on the basis of nutrient density. This is particularly true in the event of a local or national disaster. Yet, nutrient density is also critical for rebuilding the body when it is afflicted with disease. This is because disease creates the requirement for an excess of nutrients. The fact is nutritional density is the key for securing the most beneficial life-protecting—and lifesaving—value for food.

Density makes sense. In the modern world there is no room for error. In this fast paced world it is critical to gain as much power per pound from foodstuff as possible. This is particularly true in a crisis, where stress and chaos reign. The human body needs fuel to thrive. It demands the most efficient fuel possible. Plus, efficient food/fuel sources help the individual maintain strength, energy, and mental balance at a time when the world may be enveloped in turmoil (it already is). Keep calm and strong with power-packed nutrient dense foods. That is the individual's greatest advantage for superiority in difficult times.

In a crisis or high stress period it is crucial to consume food that provides the greatest nutritional value per calorie. Food must nourish the body. It must aid in satiety. In other words, it must satisfy the body's needs, physically, emotionally, and mentally. It must fuel the tissues, the organs, and the cells. It must nourish the body and in no way detract from its nourishment. In a crisis there is zero margin for error. A trendy or unscientific approach to food could prove disastrous. The foods selected in this section are guaranteed to provide the greatest density of nutrients per pound for fueling improvement of general health as well as for crisis survival.

A brief review of human physiology, as well as food chemistry, is necessary in order to comprehend nutrient density. The human body survives by converting food into energy. This process occurs continuously in every cell in the body. Human cells are capable of combusting, that is burning, three sources of fuel: carbohydrates, proteins, and fats. Only one of these is an efficient source of fuel: fat. Think about it. What was used in ancient times as fuel? It was oils such as whale blubber and olive oil, both of which were used in lamps. Today, it is crude oil that provides fuel oil and gasoline. This is the fuel humanity relies upon for survival. The same is true for the cells of the body. In contrast, wood, which is less efficient than oily fuels, is mostly carbohydrate. The fact is human cells crave fat as a source of fuel, and this issue must be thoroughly understood in the event of a crisis. There is no time for inefficiency, and in order to increase the odds for the preservation of health the individual must select food scientifically. To achieve a virtual guarantee for survival, utilize high density fuel sources, that is fatty foods, as one of the primary foodstuffs.

Protein is the second most important food, but it is not because of fuel efficiency: it is an excellent source of nutrients, particularly the all-important amino acids. A good thorough protein contains dozens of different amino acids. Protein offers dual benefits, because its amino acids can be used as fuel, but they are also needed to rebuild and repair cells, which is why this food is so essential.

Carbohydrates also serve an important role. However, with few exceptions they offer a relatively lower density of nutrients and fuel than fats/protein. Certain carbohydrate rich foods play a crucial role as a source of food, particularly for children. Plus, carbohydrates, such as wild rice, brown rice, lima beans (the best of all beans), rolled oats, dried fruit, carob molasses, and honey, are easy to feed children, plus they are well tolerated, with a low risk for allergic reactions. A few unusual carbohydrates, such as teff, amaranth, and quinoa, are highly nutritious and well digested, but they are less commonly available. Perhaps the greatest value of carbohydrates is that many of these foods are easy to store for prolonged periods: hence, the survival value of brown/wild rice, lima beans, honey, and dried fruit. What's more, they are easy to administer, especially for children and the elderly. The top quality carbohydrates for the maintenance of optimal health are listed throughout this section.

Brazil nuts

These nuts are a nutritional treasure chest. The problem is they tend to spoil. If storing, preserve in the freezer or in air tight containers. Add a natural preservative to the container, like a sprinkling of antioxidant spices: oregano, cumin, rosemary, cayenne pepper, coriander, or thyme. Or, add a few drops of oil of oregano or oil of rosemary/sage to the container. Oil of oregano is important, because Brazil nuts tend to mold, and the oregano combats food mold.

Brazil nuts are the top source of selenium. A few Brazil nuts easily provide the minimum requirement. Thus, since selenium is crucial for combating chemical or radiation poisoning, Brazil nuts may act like a sort of a life saving food/medicine to eat aggressively in the event of toxic chemical contamination. They are also one of the few dependable sources of chromium and are an excellent source of potassium and phosphorus, plus they are a top source of vitamin B_6. Furthermore, they are so rich in fatty acids for fuel and fiber that just a few Brazil nuts completely satisfy hunger.

Carob molasses

The carob tree, growing wild in the Mediterranean, may well be the manna of the Bible. While the word carob as such doesn't appear in the Bible, according to the Biblical scholar B. Montague-Drake there is no doubt that it is referred to in Luke 15:16. Carob is derived from the Arabic, "kharoub", indicating the medicinal and food value it maintained during the scientific revolution of the Islamic Empire of the Middle Ages. Then, scholars listed dozens of medicinal uses for this God-blessed plant. The fact is St. John's diet, that is the "locust and wild honey", probably did not consist of sugar coated insects; it was instead the locust bean plant, that is the wild carob pod, whose beans are to this day known as "locust beans." Have you ever seen the listing on the ingredients of processed foods, "locust bean gum?" That is an extract from the hard seeds (beans) of carob pods.

While carob powder is popular in the United States, in the Mediterranean carob is eaten as syrup or molasses. The molasses is produced by boiling the pods into a thick syrup or concentrate. What remains is a sweet easy to digest carbohydrate that is far preferable as a sweetener and/or source of food to chocolate syrup or sugar. For instance, sugar and corn syrup are pure carbohydrate, containing no nutrients, whereas carob contains a significant amount of nutrients, notably iron, calcium, and potassium.

In the Mediterranean carob molasses is used as a food rather than merely a sweetener. It makes an ideal replacement sweetener for any sugar. Its chocolate-like taste is warming and nourishing, yet, it is devoid of the typical nervous system toxicity of the cocoa bean. Use it instead of sugar on cereals. Add it as a malt-like fortifier to hot whole milk. Take a spoonful for quick energy. Carob molasses has one dependable medicinal use: it is a non-toxic, non-habit forming laxative. However, it appears to help normalize the bowels rather than induce only a temporary laxative action. Currently, researchers believe that carob, perhaps in the form of molasses, is probably the manna and certainly the "locusts/honey" of the Bible, the food that gave St. John sustenance in his missions.

To make your own locust and honey, that is protein and carbohydrate, survival food add a few nuts, milk, or cheese to carob molasses. Enjoy a treat meant for the prophets.

Fruit, dried

There is little sustenance value in dried fruit. However, it is an optimal source of naturally occurring vitamin C and bioflavonoids. In this respect it is valuable for survival. Select low sugar fruit for drying, since they contain a greater density of important nutrients than high sugar fruit such as oranges and apples. The high amount of simple sugars is detrimental, providing only hyper energy but offering little longevity nutrition. Remember, it is the nutrients in the fruit, that is the enzymes, vitamin C, folic acid, and flavonoids, that offer the greatest survival power. While sugar may be somewhat valuable as a source of energy/fuel, it is the nutrients, such as vitamin C, bioflavonoids, and carotenes, which will offer the greatest protection against disease and injury. Thus, because of its nutrient content primarily, fruit is a necessary ration and those which pack the greatest nutrient density are preferable. This is why only the most nutrient dense of all fruit are listed.

This chart lists the fruit items with the greatest nutritional density. Fruit with a high fiber content, such as papaya, pears, strawberries, and kiwi, are more filling and less caustic for individuals with blood sugar problems and/or diabetes than low fiber fruit. The most nutrient dense fruit include:

Fruit	Primary Nutrients
kiwi	folic acid, vitamin C, enzymes
papaya	folic acid, vitamin C, beta carotene, enzymes
mango	folic acid, vitamin C, beta carotene, enzymes
pears	pectin and potassium
strawberries	pectin, vitamin C, potassium, ellagic acid
blueberries	manganese, anthocyanidins
grapefruit	vitamin C, potassium, lycopene (if red)
peaches	beta carotene and potassium
apricots	beta carotene, iron, potassium
fresh pineapple	enzymes and potassium
cantaloupe	potassium, folic acid, vitamin C
watermelon	lycopene, potassium, beta carotene

Certain high sugar dried fruits are relatively high in nutrients. Apricots are exceptionally nutrient dense. They are high in sugar ,but the type they contain is readily metabolized. They are a superb source of beta carotene (and, therefore, vitamin A). What's more, they are super-rich in potassium and contain a fair amount of protein, which is unusual for a fruit. Thus, they should be a part of crisis food intake.

Always purchase dark or sulfite-free apricots. Sulfites are a type of chemical bleach used to keep apricots from turning dark colors. This chemical is a major cause of allergic reactions, and asthmatics are particularly reactive to it. Figs, another high sugar fruit, are also a tremendous source of nutrients. They pack a greater amount of calcium than any other fruit, plus they are rich in iron and potassium. Both figs and apricots are useful and convenient survival and health-giving fruit.

Herring

This is a super-rich food for survival as well as daily nutrition. This is because herring contains superb amounts of fat soluble vitamins, B vitamins, protein, and fatty acids. Two cans of herring provide a complete array of nutrients in the form of fatty vitamins, B vitamins, protein, minerals, and fuel fats, enough for an entire day—perhaps longer. The only thing it lacks is vitamin C. The fatty acids in herring are readily digested, offering fish oils, fat soluble vitamins as well as fuel calories. Herring plus dried fruit or tomatoes is a nutrient dense meal.

Honey

Honey provides fuel, that is calories, and nutrients, plus it is a lifesaving medicine. It is a relatively inexpensive natural remedy with a versatility unmatched by modern drugs. Knowing the therapeutic powers of honey is a must for those who wish to have the survival advantage for the future.

The bees use honey for food, but they also know it is a means of keeping the hive sterile. Germs cannot flourish in it. This is because of a phenomenon known as *hydroscopicity.* Honey is low in moisture. Thus, it attracts moisture. Germs are over 90% water. If a germ is deposited in honey, it is dehydrated and, therefore, dies, because the honey siphons the moisture out of it. The same occurs when pure honey is applied on the body to fight germs. It kills virtually any germ found on the tissue, usually in a matter of seconds. Honey also contains relatively large amounts of organic acids, which are natural antiseptics. Some honeys are high in hydrogen peroxide, a potent germicide. This may explain why it has been discovered that honey virtually sterilizes any wound, even those which fail to respond to antibiotics. A recent study published in the *British Journal of Surgery* found that wounds treated with honey became sterile, even those that failed to heal with antibiotic therapy. In certain instances the honey packs sterilized the wounds within a few hours. Some of these festering wounds were several years old. The honey applications cured over 80% of the wounds. However, only crude unprocessed honey exhibited this effect.

In England honey is currently used in burn wards. It is applied because it dependably sterilizes the wound, plus it speeds healing, minimizing or eliminated scarring. I have used it on burns and find it highly effective.   In contrast to other common forms of sugar, such as white sugar, brown sugar, and Karo syrup, honey is a fair source of vitamins and minerals. Dark honeys are the richest types, containing considerable amounts of potassium, magnesium, and calcium. Dr. Paavo Airola indicated that honey not only provides calcium but also aids in its absorption and retention in the body.

Wild honeys are by far the best ones medicinally. These honeys are produced by bees that visit exclusively wild medicinal plants. Such honeys are utterly rare today. Currently, only a few types are available, and all of them are harvested in a limited supply. Two examples are Wild Oregano Honey and Wild Thistle Honey. Both are extracted from beehives found in the Mediterranean mountains. In the Middle East wild raw honey is relied upon to settle upset stomach and absolve diarrhea.The honey bees that produce these rare honeys are never fed sugar. All of the honey is produced from plant nectar and sap. There is another unique type of honey made from tree blossoms, although these are only partially wild: Mediterranean Orange Blossom Honey. This honey is collected by bees, which visit the medicinal neroli or sour orange tree. The tree produces a highly aromatic nectar. Thus, the honey is also highly aromatic. These unique health enhancing honeys have never before been available in the United States. Wild Oregano and Thistle honey, as well as Mediterranean Orange Blossom Honey, are available under the brand *Wilderness Foods* (or *SuperMarket Remedies)*, which must be ordered via mail order. To order call 1-800-243-5242.

Pesticide use in the United States has essentially decimated the wild bee population. Plus, there is only minimal wild territory left in the United States. Thus, the highest quality wild honeys for internal consumption must be imported. For topical application there are a number of excellent wild or naturally created raw honeys. Any crude raw honey serves as an effective topical wound antiseptic. However, for internal use opt for the wild imported honeys if possible.

Jerky or canned meat

Have you ever wondered why the Native Americans made every effort possible to make dried meat? They knew it was among the most sustaining and nourishing of all foods and that it would help them survive difficult times, exposure to the elements, and unpredictable winters.

Jerky is one of the most nourishing of all foods, plus, if properly prepared, it lasts virtually forever. Dried meat is rich in nutrients, providing protein, vitamins, minerals, electrolytes, and fatty acids. It other words, short of vitamin C, meat contains everything necessary for survival. Meat is nourishing for another reason: it sustains the individual, more so than any other food. This is because it is rich in all eight amino acids, which are required as nourishment by every cell in the body. However, one of the main reasons meat is so essential for survival is that it provides a unique category of nutrients in a complete form: the electrolytes. These critical nutrients are required for the most essential functions of the human body. The most basic body processes, including heart nerve activity, brain/spinal nerve firing, nerve conduction, hormone production, temperature regulation, blood flow, and blood pressure are dependent upon them. These electrolytes are sodium, chloride, bicarbonate, potassium, magnesium, and iodine. Few foods contain them as a unit. Vegetables are lacking in them, as are fruit. Nuts contain a few of them, but these foods are severely lacking in sodium, iodine, and chloride. Beans are virtually devoid of these nutrients. However, meat boasts the entire category and salted meat is even more complete. Milk is the other major source.

Meat is particularly important for teenagers and growing females. A recent study published in *The Physician and Sports Medicine* (November, 1998) showed that by avoiding meat, young girls are developing severe protein and mineral deficiencies. In particular, the teenagers studied were extremely deficient in iron and zinc, and meat is the prime source of these nutrients.

Types of jerky include those made from beef, turkey, and fish. Be sure to purchase only types made without nitrates. A nitrate-free turkey jerky of excellent quality is made by Shelton's turkey farms. If making your own, be sure to add plenty of tangy spices, as these act as natural preservatives. Canned meat products in their own juices is another option.

Mackerel

A can of mackerel is so nutritious that it can help you survive for an entire day or perhaps longer. This fish is so rich in nutrients that it rapidly satisfies the appetite, providing prolonged strength and energy as well as the sensation of fullness.

Canned mackerel (with the bones) is a top source of calcium and phosphorus, both of which are needed for energy production. It is an excellent source of fuel fatty acids, plus its fatty acids aid circulation and, thus, is highly nourishing for individuals living in cold climates. Mackerel is an excellent source of B vitamins, notably pyridoxine, niacin, and biotin. It is also an excellent source of vitamin D, which is very difficult to procure in the diet. Be sure to drink the juice of the mackerel; it is rich in fat soluble vitamins as well as fish oils.

Whole milk, dried/powdered

It would be difficult to find a more useful, nutritious, and vitamin-packed food than powdered milk. The individual can essentially live on powdered milk, with a bit of vitamin C, for prolonged periods, perhaps years. It is a complete food, offering virtually every vitamin/mineral and, certainly, every amino acid needed.

It is the amino acids that are essential for survival. Without them, the organs readily degenerate. Milk is one of the few foods which offers a complete array of necessary fat, carbohydrate, and protein as well as a full array of vitamins and minerals. This is why the individual can live adequately for prolonged periods on milk supplemented with a bit of fruit and/or a crude vitamin C/flavonoid supplement such as Flavin-C. Here is an interesting confabulated food. Mix a tablespoon of Flavin-C with a pound of milk powder. To fortify it even more immensely add a tablespoon or two of Resvitanol (red sour grape powder).

Be aware that cow's milk allergy is relatively common, afflicting as many as one in three individuals. If you are allergic to milk, rely on meat, poultry, and fish as the primary source of protein.

Nuts, seeds, and nut butters

This category offers among the most nutrient dense and satisfying of all foods for survival. All nuts are useful for body sustenance. Excellent choices for nutrient density include almonds, pecans, filberts, pistachios, sunflower seeds, and Brazil nuts. However, peanuts are perhaps the most versatile, because this nut (actually legume), is the more readily digested than virtually any other type. Plus, it offers an exceptional density of certain nutrients found in lesser amounts in other nuts/legumes.

Peanuts and peanut butter

The peanut is one of the most nutrient dense foods known. It is not a true nut, instead being a legume. Certain individuals fail to tolerate legumes, and in this case other non-leguminous nuts, such as pecans, filberts, and almonds, may be preferred. However, for those who tolerate it, peanuts or peanut butter is exceptionally nutritious and easily digested. It is like a type of vegetable steak. In the form of peanut butter it keeps indefinitely. It may be preserved for even longer periods by adding antioxidant oils such as rosemary, sage, and oregano oils.

Peanuts are rich in a variety of nutrients, making them an ideal food for quick energy. They are also ideal for daily nourishment, since they pack a greater array of nutrients than virtually any other snack/food short of milk products and fresh meats. Peanuts also contain surprise components such as the flavonoid resveratrol and myoinositol. The myoinositol helps combat nerve damage and is anti-diabetic. Resveratrol is perhaps the most powerful naturally occurring anti-cancer substance known. The value of these unique naturally occurring substances in peanuts is notable. Researchers at the University of Alabama found that diabetics with nerve damage improved significantly simply by incorporating peanuts and other myoinositol-rich foods into the diet.

Peanuts are also an excellent source of vitamins and minerals, many of which are difficult to procure in the diet in large quantities. Both peanuts and peanut butter contain a high density of thiamine, niacin, pantothenic acid, and biotin as well as vitamin E, copper, and potassium. Few if any other nuts/legumes can match such nutrient density.

Aflatoxin contamination is a significant problem with peanuts/peanut butter. This danger can be ameliorated by the addition of antifungal spices, which are a particularly amenable addition to peanut butter. Simply add a few drops of oil of oregano or oil of rosemary to the peanut butter and mix thoroughly. This will halt and/or reverse mold/aflatoxin contamination.

Other nuts (mixed nuts)

All nuts offer a huge density of nutrients. Almonds, filberts, pecans, Brazil nuts, and pistachios are all top food sources. While high in fat, the type of fat they contain is incredibly healthy. A study conducted by Massachusetts researchers determined that the natural fat of nuts actually helped prevent heart attacks and had no ill effects upon the body. Nut eaters had significantly less heart attacks than those who avoid nuts.

Nuts store well, however, there is a risk they will grow mold. To help prevent this, store them in the freezer or refrigerator. Sprinkle your favorite spices or spice mixture over the nuts. You may choose to add a few drops of an antiseptic edible herbal oil to the nut container, i.e. oil of wild oregano, oil of rosemary, oil of cinnamon, oil of sage, oil of bay leaf, oil of cilantro/coriander, etc. One study found that when antioxidant spices were added to vegetable oils (nuts are a type of vegetable) the shelf life was increased as much as 900%.

Rice bran and rice polish

This is far more nourishing than any other grain-like food. Grain allergy is common. However, allergy to rice, which is a seed instead of a grain, is rather rare.

Compared to other types of bran the type from rice is high in protein. In fact, it is one of the few vegetable proteins that is nearly comparable to milk in protein value. The digestibility of rice bran protein is reportedly as high as 75%. The oils in rice bran are highly digestible. In fact, the composition is similar to that of olive oil. Rice bran oil is also high in plant sterols, which are vegetable types of cholesterol. These substances possess natural hormone like powers, and this explains the hormone balancing effects of rice bran.

Rice bran/polish are among the finest sources of natural vitamins and minerals. The types of vitamins and minerals it contains is easily absorbed. It is one of the best natural sources of natural niacin and is also exceptionally rich in pantothenic acid and biotin. Rice bran or polish is the top sources of magnesium and phosphorus in addition to supplying a good amount of manganese, potassium, and chromium.

One problem is that rice bran and polish have a limited shelf life. However, if unopened, the shelf life is at least two years.

Nutri-Sense is a supplemental source of natural rice bran and rice polish. Pure granular lecithin plus fortified ground flaxseed are added to balance the formula. Nutri-Sense is a complete formula, providing immense natural source nourishment for the body. We all need more nourishment, and Nutri-Sense provides natural source vitamins, minerals, amino acids, and fatty acids in a form which is readily absorbed. Because it is a food rather than a synthetic, Nutri-Sense has a limited shelf life and should be refrigerated after opening. However, the shelf life after opening may be extended by adding antioxidant herbal oils such as oil of sage, rosemary, oregano, and cumin.

Salmon

Canned salmon is highly nourishing for all age groups and is one of the most convenient nutrient rich foods available. It is an excellent source of amino acids, fatty acids, B vitamins, and minerals. In other words, it is a complete food.

Salmon may be regarded as sort of the nutritional cadillac of all fish. It is inordinately rich in fish oils, which offer dozens of benefits to human cellular function. Salmon is also exceptionally high in vitamins. It is one of the few fish which contains a rather complete array of B vitamins, and it is exceptionally rich in niacin, pyridoxine, and pantothenic acid. What's more, it is one of the few excellent meat sources of vitamins D and E, both of which are difficult to procure in the diet. Because it contains bones, canned salmon is one of the best supermarket sources of calcium, containing a greater amount per ounce than milk.

Alaskan wild salmon is the superior choice versus Atlantic or fresh water salmon. Wild salmon is richer in the critical essential fatty acids than the farm raised types. Wild Norwegian and Icelandic salmon are other superb choices. Salmon is one of the most nutrient dense of all foods. Rely upon it to help balance daily nutritional needs.

Sardines

This is a totally condensed food, ideal for quick nutrition. It is a meal in a can, a day's food in a tin, a survival package. Sardines possess everything required for the basic needs: amino acids, fatty acids, B vitamins, and minerals. They are also the top source of nuclear nutrients, that is RNA and DNA. Thus, with the exception of vitamin C, two or three cans of sardines provide the daily necessary ration.

Buy sardines packed in mustard, tomato sauce, or pure olive oil. Another option is sardines packed in their own fish oils, known as sild sardine oil. The latter is the most nutrient dense of all sardines, and offers a unique aromatic flavor. It is the natural sardine oils which gives this fish their intense flavor. The best sardines are made by the King Oscar company.

Unfortunately, lately I have noticed while shopping that sardines in their own oil are hard to procure. Sardines in sild oil were routinely available a few years ago. Perhaps the makers have been influenced, rather, corrupted, by the low fat craze and have halted shipment or production. With consumer persistence, the demand can be created for this preferred and nutritionally rich type of sardine so that it will be returned to the shelves.

Tuna

This is one of the most easily digested, nutritious, and filling of all foods. It is virtually pure protein with a small percentage of fat. The highest grade is white or albacore tuna, this type being richer in the all important fish oils than the regular variety. Tuna's vitamins are mainly niacin and pyridoxine, of which it is a top source. Always select tuna packed in pure water, not the oil packed varieties.

One of the great things about tuna is that when it is eaten, it fills you up. It is essentially pure protein. However, to make it even more filling pour a tablespoon or two of pure extra virgin olive oil into the container. This gives the tuna an irresistible aromatic flavor. Add to this a few chopped green onions, which provides vitamin C, and pour on vinegar for a tasty and nutritious treat.

Vegetables, dried

Vegetables offer little sustenance value for crises. They are high in moisture and low in solid nutrients such as protein, fatty acids, and vitamins. However, they are relatively high in minerals and are, of course, a top vitamin C source. Vacuum packed and/or dried vegetables have an indefinite shelf life. These types of vegetables are far more nutrient dense than the canned varieties.

Nutrient dense vegetables ideal for drying include:

- turnips
- radishes
- red and green sweet peppers
- zucchini and yellow squash
- parsley root
- parsnips
- tomatoes (actually a fruit)
- sweet or regular potatoes

Wild and brown rice

Wild rice is botanically neither rice nor grain. It is the seed of a water grass known as *Zizania aquatic*. It is one of the few items in the supermarket which may be regarded as a sort of wild organic food. Of all starches rice is perhaps the easiest to store, least likely to mold, and most nourishing. Plus, in contrast to commercial grain, it rarely causes allergic reactions.

Wild rice is an excellent source of fiber. The type it contains is soluble fiber, which means it is gentle on the gut. Researchers have found that this type of fiber helps the natural bacteria thrive, providing them with fuel. This explains why the regular consumption of wild rice greatly aids bowel function.

Wild rice is higher in certain nutrients than brown rice, notably fiber, niacin, riboflavin, silicon, phosphorus, and iron. The fact is it is several times richer in niacin and riboflavin than brown rice.

Wild and brown rice store readily. Cooked rice is highly nourishing for all age groups. Blend a 50/50 mixture of wild and brown rice and cook in mineral water. The broth remaining is extremely nourishing, being high in both B vitamins and minerals; be sure to drink it or use it as a soup base, never waste it.

Wild rice is one of the most sustaining of all types of carbohydrate sources. The protein and starch it contains are easily digested. This makes it an excellent food for children. It is also very nourishing for the elderly. Use it as the preferred grain type starch for a high level of nourishment without risk for allergy or intolerance.

Food preservatives

When a disaster strikes, the individual must be armed with methods to protect food, that is to prevent it from spoiling. Normally, refrigeration serves this purpose. It protects the food by stalling oxidation and germ growth. Yet, the possibility exists that the electricity could be disrupted and refrigeration cut off. Most individuals would regard this as a total loss, with all the food being discarded. Though this may astonish many individuals, there are measures to take which may preserve the food without refrigeration. In other words, the food doesn't have to spoil. Think about it. How did the people of ancient times, the Native Americans or the settlers of North America, keep food from spoiling? How did they manage without constantly contracting food poisoning? Now there are available substances capable of preserving food, extending the shelf life far beyond what was previously believed possible. These substances are natural antioxidants and antiseptics. If the oxidation can be blocked and germ growth halted, food may be kept virtually indefinitely, as these are the only chemical processes capable of spoiling it.

Only natural preservatives are safe for use in humans. While they are no replacement for refrigeration, if there is a disruption in common conveniences, they could prove invaluable.

Natural preservatives may be divided into two categories based upon the degree of efficacy: major and minor. Major preservatives are preferred, because of their dual action: they kill germs and halt oxidation. Minor antioxidants primarily slow oxidation and may offer a mild antiseptic action. Do not add chlorine or hydrogen peroxide to food. These are caustic chemicals capable of causing organ damage. Use only natural preservatives or antiseptics such as the following:

Major preservatives
• bee propolis
• wild oregano herb
• oil of oregano
• oil of rosemary
• oil of sage
• wild sage herb
• oil of cumin and cumin herb
• oil of bay leaf
• cloves
• salt

Add any of the above liberally to food and beverages.

Minor preservatives
• ascorbic acid — helps prevent spoilage of meat, fruit, and vegetables
• oregano herb — greatly retards food spoilage with modest but effective anti-fungal and anti-bacterial action. Halts spoilage of dry and wet foods. Great for sprinkling on fresh vegetables.
• cinnamon powder — mild antiseptic; impedes food spoilage, especially useful for meat and starches. It's antioxidant action impedes food spoilage (cinnamon oil is also highly useful)
• vitamin E — strictly an antioxidant for fats, meats, fatty foods,etc.
• red grape powder — an incredibly useful antioxidant; also blocks mold contamination.
• lemon juice — mild antiseptic; prevents fruit and vegetables from oxidizing
• vinegar — a tremendous preservative; impedes oxidation of any food; prevents microbial growth
• cayenne, black pepper, and peppercorns — mild antiseptic

Bulletin (November, 1999): Georgetown University, as well as the FDA via recent studies at the University of Tennessee, have proven that oil of oregano kills germs in food, on food, and in tissue culture. Defeated germs killed included Candida albicans, staph, Listeria, yeasts, molds, Yersinia, E. coli, and even pseudomonas.

CHAPTER 4

Wilderness Foods

The purpose of this section is to share my personal knowledge of wilderness foods. Only a finite percentage of Americans are capable of foraging for food. First, it is virtually impossible to procure enough food from foraging. The energy it takes to collect the food is greater than the energy the food will provide. However, it is reasonable to presume that certain industrious individuals are capable of finding food outside of supermarkets and health stores. The key is to realize what could realistically be foraged. In other words, in this section you will learn what are the wild or rural foods you can find without herculean efforts.

I frequently forage. It is a relaxing hobby. I do most of my foraging while on trips in remote regions, where the items I pick are relatively free of pollution. Yet, I also frequent berry bushes or trees within a few miles of my home. Remember, sun-ripened wild fruit is always superior nutritionally to the commercial varieties. Foraging is a healthy hobby, if you know what to look for. When foraging, beware of one major enemy: ticks. Be sure to check the body for ticks after any wilderness jaunt.

The greatest problem is that there is little wild food available. The exceptions are rather remote regions, such as the woods of Northern California, Oregon, Washington State, Minnesota, Michigan, and Maine as well as certain Appalachian

83

states, where individuals are accustomed to foraging. In Canada foraging is realistic, especially in the regions of lakes and forests in the far north. Thus, perhaps 5% of the North American population live in regions ideal for foraging. However, for the other 95% a few industrious individuals could procure food, perhaps through hunting and fishing. In rural regions there may be a plethora of wild foods such as wild asparagus, berries, and various edible animals. Yet, even in the wide open space of America's rural regions feeding a family from the wild would be extremely arduous, perhaps impossible. Note that the American Indians were readily exterminated simply by disrupting access to their normal food production/hunting procedures. If the natives failed to survive at the turn of the century in the wilderness, how realistic is it that massive amounts of Americans could do so? The fact is only the most astute, knowledgeable, and savvy individual could successfully feed off the wild without the support of the commercialized convenience world. Because of these factors, only the most rudimentary wild edible substances, which are highly accessible to relatively large numbers of individuals, are important. In other words, the foods in this section are selected, because they are familiar to nearly everyone and, thus, the majority of individuals can apply this information rapidly, without becoming an herb expert. Plus, there can be no chance for confusion with non-edible or even poisonous plants. Thus, everyone, from small children to the elderly, can safely follow the advice in this section.

Perhaps of greatest significance is the fact that these wild plants can be procured to add nutrition to the daily menu. Wild foods are far richer in vitamins and minerals than commercial foods. For instance, wild dandelion greens may contain as much as five times more vitamin A (as beta carotene) than greenhouse-grown varieties, and, in addition, up to ten times the potassium levels.

Dandelion greens

These are not difficult to find. They are right in your lawn. They are most edible during the spring and early summer. The best greens are the young leaves, which may grow under the older leaves. Older leaves are fibrous and inedible, that is they are mostly cellulose. Be sure the dandelion greens you pick are from an area not sprayed with pesticides.

Dandelions are extremely rich in nutrients, far richer than any vegetable you can buy. They are extremely high in beta carotene as well as vitamin C. For B vitamins they pack a greater density of riboflavin and niacin than any common vegetable. They contain a legion of life-saving minerals, particularly iron, calcium, phosphorus, magnesium, and potassium. What's more, they provide both protein and essential fatty acids.

Dandelion greens are highly protective for the body's most critical organs: the liver and kidneys. In Germany they are relied upon for liver cleansing, while in France they are highly touted as a natural diuretic. Simply pick the greens, wash thoroughly, and cook or eat raw. Sprinkle with lemon juice or red grape powder if desired. Dandelion greens are a complete food.

Fishing

This is one of the easiest types of all foraging. Virtually everyone knows how to fish. The nice thing about fishing is that anything you catch is edible as long as it is from relatively unpolluted water. Prepare basic fishing gear with reliable artificial lures just in case food sources run scarce. Remember, bait, such as worms, amphibians, and insects, can always be found.

To catch fish, everyone knows that the proper gear is required. Yet, the most important component is neither hook, line, nor sinker— it is belief. You must believe you will catch fish; you must be confident. They are there, and they are hungry. You must know this. Believe you will catch them, and you shall. This is more important than any gadget or technique.

Fishing is a relaxing, enjoyable hobby, plus it may provide valuable nutrition for the table. Nothing supercedes the taste of freshly caught fish. Be sure to cook your catch in spices, which offer both the benefit of great flavor plus stimulation of digestion.

Apples, pears, plums, and peaches

There are millions of wild trees (or abandoned orchards) bearing tasty fruit, although the produce may not appear as lovely as that in the grocery store. Be sure to remove fruit from only public or wilderness land. Don't enter private orchards without permission. If you desire food, simply ask. Most growers are generous with excess produce. Note: pears are one of the most readily digested of all fruit; an entire family can virtually live off of a well endowed pear tree for several days, perhaps weeks.

Mulberries

Virtually every block in the northern United States has within it a mulberry tree or perhaps a child who can find one. The mulberry may be the top survival berry. This is because it is high in a special chemical that helps reverse virtually any type of poisoning: resveratrol. Plus, mulberries are a good source of vitamin C and potassium, which are also needed for detoxification.

Don't wait for a disaster to strike to collect mulberries. This is one of the most nutrient rich of all berries, available to virtually everyone. These sun-enriched berries are far more nourishing than the rather bland nutrient poor varieties found in the supermarkets. Plus, mulberries offer significant anti-toxic and anti-cancer powers. If you pick an excess, they may be dried in the sun or in an oven under low heat. This way you can eat them continuously.

Wild strawberry leaves and berries

This exotic plant, rare today, once filled the meadows, forests, and clearings of virtually every Eastern, Southern, and Midwestern state in the country. It grew like a weed. Native Americans filled baskets full of this fragrant fruit, devouring it as an exotic treat. The leaves of the wild strawberry plant were respected by the primitives for anti-diarrheal powers. The medicinal power of wild strawberry leaves is largely due to its high content of tannic acids. The berries are rare currently, unless the individual lives in the remote reaches of Canada, Montana, Michigan, Minnesota, Maine, and Alaska. They may also be found in the wild meadows of Nebraska. The fresh leaves are super-rich in vitamin C.

Strawberry leaf tea is one of the most nourishing of all beverages. Fortunately, this is commercially available as *WildPower Tea*. Brew this tea and add hot milk and honey for a pleasant flavonoid rich drink. This was the brew that saved George Washington and his men from dying of scurvy at Valley Forge. Native Americans taught them to dig beneath the snow to discover the leaves, still green and vitamin/flavonoid rich.

Drink *WildPower Tea* for a taste of an original, nourishing Native American formula. It is highly refreshing and makes a perfect evening hot drink or daytime cool beverage.

Wild blueberries and huckleberries

Once found in dozens of states, these beautiful berries are extremely nourishing, exotic in taste, and even filling. They are more rare now and only found in remote areas such as in the wilderness regions of Northern California, Washington state, Oregon, Michigan, Northern Minnesota, Northern Wisconsin, Alaska, and Maine.

These berries' richest component is a group of chemicals called anthocyanidins, the substances responsible for their brilliant color. The anthocyanidins are potent cancer fighters, plus they aid vision, a fact which explains the visually endowed bears' preference for them. Wild blueberries are an excellent source of potassium and a good source of vitamin C. The leaves are also nutritious, being high in vitamin C, flavonoids, and potassium. Add the leaves to hot water and let steep; the tea is a reliable cure for diarrhea as well as diabetes.

Wild raspberries and blackberries

These are the most abundant of all wild berries and are particularly ubiquitous in Midwestern states as well as the East Coast. They are found nearly everywhere in Canada. Thus, they are one of the easiest of all wild foods to procure. Wild raspberries/blackberries are a good source of vitamin C and are super-rich in flavonoids. The leaves and berries of these plants are excellent digestive aids and are curative for mild diarrhea. Raspberry leaf tea is a dependable aid for female complaints, particularly menstrual discomfort or excessive menstrual bleeding.

Wild grapes, grape shoots, and grape leaves

Wild grapes are rarely used by Americans, yet they are perhaps the most ubiquitous of all wild berries. All parts of the plant are edible. The young shoots or curls are a top source of vitamin C and are pleasantly tart in taste. However, the grapes themselves are super high in the vitamin. The leaves, that is the young ones, are entirely edible, either raw or soaked in vinegar water. They too are an excellent source of vitamin C as well as resveratrol. While extremely tart, the grapes are a great source of vitamins, minerals, and flavonoids. A handful of wild grapes provides the minimum daily need for vitamin C and potassium. They ripen in late August and September.

Rose hips

These can be found everywhere, even in flower gardens and parks. However, the best ones come from wild rose bushes, which are also prolific. Rose hips are the best source of vitamin C of any North American plant. They are edible primarily after the first few frosts. They may be dried and immersed into boiling water; this helps extract the vitamin C. They are also rich in protein, essential fatty acids, and vitamin E, the latter being found in the hard seeds lodged within the pulp. Rose hips are also a mineral concentrate, providing large amounts of iron, phosphorus, and potassium.

If you have access to the wilderness, gather rose hips after the first frosts. Dry them and store in the freezer. Add the dried hips to any herbal tea or grind them and add to soups or sauces. Fortify your food through the addition vitamin C- and flavonoid-rich wild rose hips. Your health will improve as a result.

Nuts

Virtually everyone has made at least one attempt to collect nuts from the wild. The most common wild nut trees are black walnuts, hickory nuts, hazelnuts, butternuts, and pecans. Extracting the nuts from their shells is arduous. However, the meats are delicious and highly nourishing. If there is no food to be found, locate nut trees and fill bags full. This will provide dense nourishment for survival, especially in the event of the onset of difficult winters. Nut oils provide the perfect fuel for the cells of the body in combating cold temperature. Plus, nuts are an excellent source of essential fatty acids, so direly needed for the health of the hair, skin, and nails. Thus, a handful of wild or plantation nuts provides immense nutritional support, especially for combating the ill effects of cold weather.

Other wilderness foods

There are hundreds of other foods which may be harvested from the wild or from public lands. This chapter is merely an attempt to guide individuals to the most prolific and easily accessible of these. Perhaps the individual could add to this list significantly with certain items of favorite wild nourishment. Wild asparagus, onions, garlic, chicory, lamb's quarters, yellow dock, sumac berries, rice—the list is endless.

Chapter 5
The Illnesses

There are tens of thousands of illnesses which afflict humankind; no book can cover them all. However, the purpose of this book is to cover those illnesses which will commonly occur during human difficulties or crises and which are most likely to cause discomfort, disability, disease, and even death in the event of human catastrophe. The attempt here is to select the most common illnesses that will pose problems. It is to provide help in the event medical care either falters or is not accessible.

The conditions are listed alphabetically to allow for the quickest possible reference. Plus, the objective is to use the most simple terms possible, ones that the average individual would readily recognize. For instance, instead of using the medical term gastritis "Stomachache/pain", is listed, which is the common terminology. Instead of cervical strain, "Stiff/painful neck" is listed. Plus, treatments are constructed with a priority towards crisis management. Yet, they can also be applied to the treatment of chronic disease. Thus, instead of listing "arthritis," which is a chronic disease and is usually not a crisis, "Joint pain" is listed. However, the information under joint pain is useful to the arthritic. What's more, within many of the listings the most common and easy to recognize signs and symptoms have also been established. This is so the condition may be readily diagnosed.

Here is the objective: to provide the individual with the most powerful, versatile, and simple to use remedies available. In an emergency there is no time to think; only to react. This book gives you the tools to react properly to difficult or dangerous situations.

Whether for everyday disasters, chronic health problems, toxic chemical exposure, or acts of Nature, the individual needs a quick reference to determine what to do. This chapter serves precisely this function.

Unless otherwise mentioned all amounts listed represent adult dosages. For children or tiny individuals reduce the amount by at least half or perhaps two thirds.

Abdominal pain

The problem with abdominal pain is that it might be a mild incident amenable to simple measures, yet, it could also be a medical or surgical emergency. There are circumstances where sudden abdominal pain is non-surgical. For instance, pancreatitis, that is inflammation of the pancreas, causes severe abdominal pain, but surgery is rarely required. While sudden abdominal pain is virtually always a medical emergency requiring immediate physician supervision, in a disaster it may be impossible to procure medical or surgical care. In other words, the hospitals and doctors' offices may themselves be disabled or destroyed.

Methods of combat against abdominal pain
• Seek medical care immediately. Give no food or drink: only pure water at most.
• Keep the individual warm; cover with blankets if possible. Lay the individual on his/her right side.
• Rub essential oils on the body, but avoid harsh touching or pushing on the abdomen; gentle rubbing to apply the oils is

allowed. Rub the oils on the back, face, and neck as well as the soles of the feet. Concentrate on rubbing the spine, buttocks, and feet. Repeat the essential oil rub often. The best oils for this purpose are pure wild oil of oregano, oil of lavender, Oil of Bay Berry, oil of rosemary, and oil of sage.

• oil of ginger (emulsified in extra virgin olive oil) should be the first substance to consume. If tolerated, it will greatly ease the internal organs and combat stomach/intestinal distress. Take 2 or more drops twice daily under the tongue or in a small amount of water.

• Take wild oil of oregano, as researched by Georgetown University, the type emulsified in extra virgin olive oil . The safest method is to avoid taking anything into the stomach. Thus, take the oil under the tongue, one or two drops as often as necessary to halt the pain. In severe abdominal pain this may induce vomiting. However, the vomiting itself may be therapeutic. Often, this safe edible herbal oil will halt the pain rapidly, perhaps within minutes. This remedy may prove lifesaving in case medical care is arrested.

• If food/beverage can be taken by mouth, begin with simple remedies that relax the digestive tract. Make tea from fresh ginger root. This is soothing and pain relieving. Oil of fennel and rosemary are also highly relaxing to the gut. Add a few drops in hot water or juice and sip until pain is relieved. Remember, significant abdominal pain unrelieved by simple remedies requires immediate medical attention.

• If supplements can be taken by mouth, try BromaZyme and/or HerbSorb. Both are well tolerated and are highly effective in reversing digestive disorders and/or pain.

Special Note: in this and all subsequent illnesses described in this book several natural cures are listed.

Things to avoid

• don't eat anything for at least 24 hours, in other words, rest the gut until the individual improves. At most, drink pure water or perhaps eat a small amount of raw honey.

• don't take aspirin or other anti-pain/anti-inflammation drugs.

Aching feet

No one can afford to suffer with aching or tired feet. Revitalize the feet with essential oils. Rubbed topically, the oils quickly ease foot pain. They are also well absorbed from the porous skin of the feet, invigorating the entire body. Burning of the feet may warn of vitamin deficiency, notably a lack of vitamin B_5 (pantothenic acid).

Aching feet combat kit

• Oil of Bay Berry — rub on feet vigorously.
• oil of oregano — rub on soles of feet. Also, take 2 drops twice daily in juice or water.
• oil of lavender — rub on soles of feet as desired.
• pantothenic acid (500 mg capsules) — take 1 or 2 capsules twice daily.

AIDS

The problem with AIDS is that virtually anyone, no matter what is his/her status, can become infected with this frequently fatal infestation. Thus, an infected individual may, if injured, liberate the germ in secretions or blood, and whoever comes in contact may become infected. This is how most health workers contract the disease. However, this mode of transmission is comparatively rare. The vast majority of individuals develop AIDS from sex. Obviously, IV drug abuse is the other major cause. With this disease the individual is essentially a cess pool of infection.

In a crisis setting individuals may come in contact with blood from injury victims. It is crucial to protect yourself from such a potential disaster, since AIDS is largely transmitted by blood.

AIDS combat kit

• oil of oregano — rub on any open wound or region which may be infected by the virus or which is contaminated by human blood. Also, take 2 or more drops under the tongue three times daily. For full blown AIDS use the SuperStrength, 2 or 3 drops under the tongue three times daily plus 10 to 20 drops twice daily in juice or water.
• oil of rosemary — take 10 drops twice daily.
• oil of cumin — take 10 drops twice daily.

- oil of edible cinnamon — take 5 to 10 drops twice daily.
- organic selenium — take 400 mcg daily.
- Oregamax — take 8 or more capsules daily.

Foods that help
- protein rich foods, such as fresh meat, nuts, whole milk products, yogurt, fermented soy, and fish, are invaluable, since this is a protein/tissue wasting disease.
- garlic, onion, leeks, cinnamon (contain anti-viral compounds)
- raw almonds (as a source of protease inhibitors)

Allergic reactions
Allergic reactions plague modern humanity. For instance, as many as 1 in 3 Americans have food allergies to such a degree that they suffer with daily symptoms. It is significant enough to be allergic to certain foods, but the problem today is that we are being exposed to tens of thousands of synthetic chemicals, all of which can provoke allergic reactions. Some of the most pervasive of these allergy causing chemicals include MSG, sulfites, Aspartame, saccharin, and food dyes.

There are hundreds of symptoms due to allergy. Some of the main symptoms include:
- hives or other sudden rashes
- shortness of breath and/or swelling in the throat
- sinus attacks
- itchy skin
- urinary discomfort
- headaches
- irritable bowel
- heartburn/indigestion
- diarrhea
- bloating after eating
- fatigue
- mood swings and/or irritability
- depression

Hives are one of the major signs of allergic reactions. If you develop them, it is a signal that your body is reacting to something you have ingested, either a food or a drug.

Allergic reaction combat kit
• oil of oregano — take 2 or more drops under the tongue twice daily; also, take 5 drops as frequently as necessary in juice or water.
• Oregamax capsules — take 2 or more capsules several times daily.
• Royal Kick premium grade royal jelly (unless allergic to bee stings) — take 4 capsules three or more times daily.
• organic selenium — take 200 mcg every 8 hours until symptoms abate. Then, take 200 to 400 mcg daily.
• pantothenic acid (capsules, not hard tablets) — take 500 mg three or more times daily.
• BromaZyme – take 2 or 3 capsules several times daily until the reaction is eliminated.

Things to avoid
• synthetic food dyes and artificial flavorings
• processed food
• drugs, including antibiotics
• NutraSweet and saccharin

Angina (see also Heart attack)
This is heart pain, which is believed to be caused by a lack of oxygen to the heart muscle. Yet, it is closely correlated with mental stress, especially anger and hostility. Relaxation and peace of mind is the antithesis of this condition. Put simply, if your heart muscle hurts, your inner heart, that is your soul, also hurts.

The role of hostility in the cause of heart disease was recently confirmed by medical science. Researchers publishing in the *American Journal of Cardiology* determined that hostility and anger specifically damage the arteries of the heart, the very ones responsible for preventing angina.

Technically, angina is a type of pain that occurs over the left side of the upper chest, i.e. over the heart, which may spread to areas of what are known as referred pain. The nerves to the heart interconnect to other regions like the jaw, left side of the arm, upper back, and neck. This is why anginal pain may strike any of these regions. Much of the pain may be related to a deficiency of oxygen. In other words, the arteries supplying the heart are diseased and fail to deliver sufficient oxygen, resulting in chest pain.

Physical disorders play a primary role in this condition. The arteries of the heart may be narrowed. The blood is often too thick, impeding oxygen/nutrient delivery. Also, the hormonal system may be disrupted, especially if the individual is under stress. What's more, dietary factors play an enormous role. Smoking and alcohol consumption greatly aggravate this condition. To correct the angina procure a thorough evaluation by a physician (hopefully one with a nutritional orientation), and take the following remedies:

Angina combat kit
• oil of rosemary — 5 drops under the tongue several times daily during an attack; as a regular amount, take 5 to 10 drops daily.
• oil of oregano — take 2 drops under the tongue as often as necessary.
• Juice of Rosemary — as a circulatory tonic, take 2 or more ounces daily.
• red grape powder (to regenerate the arteries) — take 4 capsules three times daily.
• bromelain (uncoated) — take 3 capsules three times daily on an empty stomach (BromaZyme is a powerful and excellent choice.)

Foods that help
• squash, pumpkin, zucchini, and yellow squash
• garlic, onions, leek, shallots
• nuts and seeds

Things to avoid
• caffeine, chocolate, iced tea
• alcoholic beverages and beer
• nitrated/processed meats
• cigarette, cigar, and pipe smoke
• stress, hostility, anger, and apathy

Anthrax

This is a severe acute disease caused by a bacteria called *B. anthracis*. It usually occurs on farms, but urban outbreaks are a possibility. There have been no *major* outbreaks of this disastrous illness in recent history, but there have been outbreaks. In Ontario (1998) dozens of individuals contracted this condition in its less fatal form, that is the type that attacks the skin. In the United States during 1998 there were numerous incidents of purported anthrax spore releases, mostly in public buildings. All were false alarms.

Exposure to anthrax spores is nearly always fatal. The problem is that when the spores are inhaled in large numbers, the germs multiply rapidly in the lungs, suffocating the individual. It is the weapon of germ warfare. Thus, there is no medical defense.

An outbreak of anthrax remains a significant possibility, especially since the development of active infection in Canada. in 1998. While antibiotics are useful for the skin manifestations, they offer no certain protection in the event of spore release. Thus, the individual must rely upon natural remedies as an adjunct. The fact is natural cures, particularly the edible essential oils, would prove lifesaving in the event of an anthrax outbreak.

Anthrax combat kit

• oil of oregano SuperStrength — apply topically to skin lesions. If spore contamination/lung infection occurs, massive amounts will be needed, like 40 to 80 drops daily in juice or water. Also, take a few drops under the tongue as often as every five minutes.
• oil of cumin — take 10 to 20 drops daily in juice or water.
• oil of bay leaf — take 10 to 20 drops daily in juice or water.
• oil of lavender — use topically on lesions.
• raw garlic/onion — consume as much as possible
• Black seed-plus — take 3 capsules four times daily.
• protective mask and clothing (plasticized jackets/suits, gloves, etc.)

Foods that help

• raw onion juice — a cup twice daily
• raw wild oregano honey — 6 or more tablespoons daily

Arsenic poisoning

Heavy metal poisoning is one of the modern world's most monumental disasters. This occurs largely in industrial workers, yet, it can also develop in unwitting victims, who live near pollution generating industrial complexes.

Poisoning by arsenic is far from remote. This heavy metal is a component of a variety of industrial chemicals, notably insecticides, fumigants, weed killers, fruit sprays, and rodent poisons. The highly toxic arsenic gas is transported every day on the railways and roads of North America. As a result of its rather ubiquitous nature thousands of cases of chronic arsenic poisoning occur every year. Symptoms of arsenic poisoning include:

- metallic taste in the mouth
- numbness and tingling in the nerves
- odd skin lesions, which are dry and excoriated
- muscular weakness and/or paralysis
- confusion
- headaches, usually chronic
- burning sensation in the limbs
- nausea and vomiting
- loss of appetite
- weight loss
- vague abdominal pain
- petechiae (tiny skin hemorrhages)
- watery diarrhea (may be severe and prolonged)

Arsenic detoxification kit

- organic selenium — take 200 mcg three times daily.
- calcium and magnesium — take 1200 mg of calcium and 600 mg of magnesium daily. Do not use magnesium oxide. It is poorly absorbed and usually causes diarrhea if taken in large amounts.
- oil of cumin — take 10 to 20 drops twice daily. If exposure is severe, double or triple this amount.
- oil of rosemary (strong liver and nerve protection) — take 20 drops twice daily. If exposure is severe, double this amount.
- oil of cilantro/coriander — take 10 to 20 drops twice daily. If exposure is severe, double or triple this amount.

- NAC (N-acetyl cysteine) — 1000 mg daily.
- zinc chelate — 75 to 100 mg daily.
- red grape powder — take 2 capsules three times daily.

Aspergillus infection (Aspergillosis)

This is a potentially devastating infection by a bizarre fungi (mold), which lives primarily in soil. This fungus was once thought only to attack weakened or immune compromised individuals. Yet, today relatively healthy individuals are developing the infection.

Aspergillus is known as a filamentous fungus, meaning it grows in tiny filaments or threads. These threads can invade virtually any tissue in the body, but they have a preference for attacking the sinuses, lungs, and heart valves. However, they also readily invade the skin, nails, external ear, nasal mucosa, vagina, and even the bone marrow. Cancer patients are its greatest victims. Globally, some 300,000 cancer patients die yearly from aspergillosis, candidiasis, and other fungal infections.

There is a virtual disaster occurring in America regarding this germ. According to bone marrow transplant expert Dr. Elias Anaissie aspergillus is invading individuals from a ubiquitous source: drinking water. He describes how tap water is loaded with the fungus, explaining that "chlorine doesn't touch aspergillus." He is so concerned about this that he recommends hospitalized patients receive sponge baths instead of showers, which aerosolize the germ. Scientific studies confirm Dr. Anaissie's concerns: simply turning on a sink can liberate enough aspergillus in the air that it can be detected six feet away.

While there are no drugs which destroy this germ, Nature provides the answer. Oil of oregano decimates it. As described by European researchers as little as a tenth of a percent concentration (a drop or two in a few ounces of water), halts and prevents its growth. A mere one percent concentration obliterates it.

Aspergillus infection combat kit

- oil of oregano (SuperStrength is best) — take 2 to 5 drops three times daily under the tongue. Take 5 to 10 drops twice daily in juice or water. Note: also rub the oil of oregano around sinus region and nose or place a small amount on a Q-tip and apply in nose (for sinus/lung fungus). Before drinking add a drop or more of oil of oregano to any suspect water.

- Oregamax capsules — take at least 3 capsules twice daily. For stubborn cases take 3 capsules three times daily.
- Resvitanol — take 3 capsules twice daily.
- black seed capsules (Black seed-plus) — take 3 capsules twice daily. **Note**: aspergillus infection may cause symptoms which mimic the common cold.

Things to avoid
- refined sugar, wheat products, rye products, wheat grass
- chlorinated tap water

Asthma

This is one of the gravest epidemics facing the American public, because despite medical care the death rate from this disease has nearly doubled. As many as 1 in 15 individuals in North America have asthma, an incredibly high number. Yet, for asthmatic victims the greatest desperation results because of the fact that the medical profession offers no cure for this potentially disastrous illness. It is ironic that an orthodox medical journal, *Hippocrates Magazine*, states "there is no cure for asthma." This is despite the fact that Hippocrates himself, working in the 5th century B.C., apparently cured it with herbs.

Mold allergy and/or infection is the most likely cause for today's asthma epidemic. It is a condition rarely suspected or diagnosed by physicians. Molds are also an indirect cause. They poison the immune system, leaving it vulnerable to attack by viruses. Other major factors include chemical sensitivity, air pollution, food allergy, and immunization reactions. Common symptoms of asthma include:
- chest tightness
- wheezing
- coughing
- inability to take a clear deep breath
- inability to exhale completely
- sensitivity to chemicals, fumes, and odors

Asthma Combat Kit

• oil of oregano — take 2 or more drops under the tongue twice or more daily.
• wild oregano herb (Oregamax capsules) — take 2 or 3 capsules twice daily.
• black seed capsules (Black seed-plus) — take 2 or more capsules three times daily.
• Flavin-C – take 3 capsules twice daily.
• oil of rosemary – take 5 to 10 drops twice daily in juice or water.

Things to Avoid

• tartrazine (Yellow dye #5) and other synthetic food dyes
• MSG and sulfites
• white sugar

Athlete's foot and/or jock itch

These aggravating unrelenting conditions afflict tens of millions of North Americans. Every manner of cream, powder, and formula is applied to the feet/groin in attempt to cure it. Yet, it is easy to eradicate. Athlete's foot is caused by a fungus, which invades and feeds off the superficial layers of skin on the feet. This fungus eats keratin, the protein which makes up skin. It also feeds off of sugar, which is delivered to the skin from the blood. It is usually contracted from moist contaminated public places such as school showers, gymnasiums, bathtubs, and bathroom floors. Jock itch is caused by the same fungus.

Athlete's foot/jock itch combat kit

• oil of oregano — rub on feet, morning and night. For jock itch dilute (three to five drops in a teaspoon of myrtle or olive oil).
Apply once or twice daily. Also, take 2 or 3 drops under the tongue twice daily.
• crushed raw garlic in olive oil (could be irritating) — apply at night due to the odor. Note: this may lead to a garlic odor throughout the body.

Things to avoid
• don't go barefoot in public places
• synthetic socks, which retain moisture and germs (use cotton or wool instead)
• white sugar and sweets feed the fungus, making eradication difficult

Back pain

Back pain and injury are perhaps the most common causes of disability in the United States today. In a crisis back pain is an utter disaster. Who can afford to be crippled at a time of difficulty?

Many of the drugs which fight pain are caustic to the stomach and intestines. Thus, their unsupervised use may cause more harm than good. This is why it is more appropriate to rely on natural remedies to combat disaster-related pain. Use home remedies combined with appropriate exercise to rebuild the back and eliminate the pain.

Back pain combat kit
• bromelain (uncoated capsules, i.e. BromaZyme) — take 2 to 4 capsules three times daily on an empty stomach.
• oil of oregano (SuperStrength is the best) — rub topically on painful region. Take 5 to 10 drops twice daily in juice or water.
• red grape powder — take a teaspoon twice daily in juice or water.
• Flavin-C — take 3 capsules twice daily.

Foods that help
• raw almonds
• fresh papaya including seeds
• cayenne pepper, oregano, and sage

Other ideas
• don't sleep on the stomach; preferably, sleep on the right side
• squat low before lifting heavy objects; lift with hips and thighs
• don't eat foods to which you are allergic

Bed Sores and other skin ulcers

Bed sores are open wounds that afflict primarily the elderly and infirm. They are caused largely by constant pressure against the tissues, the result of immobility. These sores notoriously fail to heal despite aggressive medical treatment, which includes massive antibiotic therapy and surgical debridement.

Varicose ulcers, also known as stasis ulcers, are similar to bed sores in appearance. They are due to poor blood flow as a result of sluggish venous return. In other words, the blood stagnates in the lower extremities, leading to infection and/or ulceration. A history of varicose veins increases the risk, as does diabetes and atherosclerosis.

Because their circulation is so poor, diabetics frequently develop ulcerations in the extremities, particularly in the legs and feet. The ulcers easily become infected, which may lead to gangrene.

Medical treatment for bed sores usually fails. What's more, repeated dosages of antibiotics damage the immune system, causing deep seated fungal infections, both in the wound(s) and internal organs. This is why yeasts are frequently cultured from these wounds, although they are usually regarded as a source of "secondary infection."

Fungi thrive on diseased and/or dead tissue. In a forest molds and mushrooms do not grow on healthy trees. They grow prolifically on diseased, dying, or dead trees. In other words, fungi attack the sick and debilitated. The same applies to human tissues. This is why they attack chronic wounds.

Oil of oregano, as well as other essential oils, such as rosemary, myrtle, and lavender oils, are the agents of choice for the topical treatment of bed sores, varicose ulcers, and diabetic ulcers. Oil of oregano in particular exhibits both antibacterial and antifungal activity. It is ideal for use on open wounds, since it penetrates deep into injured tissue and coats both healthy and diseased portions. It helps sterilize the wound and its secretions. It disperses pus. Plus, it helps speed the healing of these difficult to cure wounds.

Oil of oregano is the first choice for bed sores or other poorly healing open wounds. It should be utilized topically as well as internally. Usually, only small amounts are needed topically. Other oils may be of even greater value for speeding healing, notably the oils of rosemary, myrtle, lavender, and bay berry. The oils can be administered simultaneously with medical therapy. They should routinely be applied on open wounds which are being treated with systemic antibiotics. If the wound is too sensitive, rub the oils on the surrounding skin. This speeds healing, eradicates infection, and prevents further infection from developing.

Oregano oil's superiority over antibiotics lies largely in its potent action against fungi. Fungi are parasites; in other words, they are opportunists. They invade weakened and diseased tissues. Healthy tissue is immune to them.

If the infection is destroyed, open sores heal rapidly. In other words, it is the infection which is delaying the healing. Nutritional deficiency may also play a role, as a lack of vitamins A, C, B_5, B_6, and essential fatty acids greatly impede wound healing, as do deficiencies of zinc, iron, and selenium· Merely replacing the deficient nutrients greatly accelerates wound healing.

Skin ulcerations must be regarded seriously, especially in the chronically ill. In diabetics open wounds may proceed to more serious conditions: gangrene and amputation. If the infection can be rapidly eliminated, the wound will heal quickly, and the crisis will be resolved.

Bed sore/open wound combat kit
• oil of oregano — apply topically as often as needed and take internally, 5 to 10 drops twice daily. Rub on skin surrounding the wound. To accelerate wound healing apply honey over the oregano oil.
• crude raw honey — apply topically on wound site and cover.
• Oil of Bay Berry — for wound healing; apply as needed; rub on skin surrounding the wound.
• oil of lavender — for wound healing; apply as needed directly to wound or on surrounding skin.
• Flavin-C — for stimulating cartilage and skin regeneration; take 3 capsules twice daily.
• pantothenic acid — for stimulating wound healing; take 500 mg twice daily.

- zinc chelate — take 75 to 100 mg daily until wound heals.
- selenium — take 300 to 600 mcg daily until wound heals.

Bee Stings (see also Killer Bees)

About 1 in 200 people is severely allergic to bee stings. Yet, every individual is vulnerable to suffering from the painful stings of these creatures. What's more, there is a new threat, the killer bees, which can cause fatality in virtually anyone, allergic or not.

Bee stings are the most common type of insect bite in the Northern United States and Canada. In the Southeast fire ants are the primary stinging insect. Repeated stings by fire ants make the individual more vulnerable to bee sting hypersensitivity. Conversely, individuals sensitive to bee stings are usually highly sensitive to fire ant stings.

For the vast majority of individuals bee stings are easy to resolve. Simply apply an antivenom herb extract to the sting site. The best antivenom herbs are oil of oregano, juice of raw garlic, and juice of raw onion. Oil of oregano is perhaps the most aggressive and potent of these. However, if this is unavailable, simply crush raw garlic or onion. Apply the maceration to the sting site. Eradication of pain and swelling should be immediate. For those with severe reactions the therapy should be more aggressive; call for medical help immediately. Symptoms of life-threatening bee sting shock include:
- hives
- throat tightness
- inability to talk (swollen vocal cords)
- inability to swallow
- coughing spasms and/or wheezing
- weakness and/or dizziness
- loss of consciousness
- severe swelling at the sting site

If any of these symptoms develop, seek medical care immediately. However, edible oil of oregano is an absolute lifesaver in this scenario, as is demonstrated by the following:

> *Case history:* Mr. J. was vacationing in Vale, Colorado, when his worst nightmare occurred: he was stung in the neck by a bee. The problem is Mr. J. is highly allergic to bee stings, and just a few months prior he nearly died from a sting. Rapidly, he developed a severe toxic reaction; his neck swelled up enormously, and he collapsed almost immediately. Fortunately, an herbalist was in his presence. This brave soul grabbed his bottle of oil of oregano (North American Herb & Spice Co.), placed several drops in Mr. J.'s mouth and rubbed it on his neck. Within minutes Mr. J. was revived; his neck swelling was halted, in fact, it was reversed. By the time the ambulance arrived he was completely well and did not require further care. This immensely valuable herbal substance, that is the wild oil of oregano, saved his life.

What to do in a bee sting emergency:

Get medical help immediately, and:
• remove the stinger if possible
• saturate the sting site with oil of oregano or garlic/onion maceration
• for severe toxic/systemic reactions give oil of oregano by mouth (only use the edible kind by North American Herb & Spice: do not use aromatherapy oregano oil and cheap imitations internally)
• apply ice to the wound if the swelling fails to recede
• seek medical care if necessary (or available)

Bee sting combat kit
• oil of oregano — apply this life-saving oil directly to the sting site. Repeat as needed. The oil also helps dislodge the stinger.
• garlic cloves — crush and apply maceration to the wound (not necessary if oil of oregano is available).
• raw onion bulb — crush and apply juice and/or maceration to the wound.
• tweezers (for removing the stinger)

Killer bee combat kit (see also Killer Bees)
Same as the aforementioned, however:
• if the bees are still attached, pour oregano oil on them; this will kill them or drive them off. If a spray bottle is handy, add the oregano oil to it; pump spray the bees. Oil of cumin may also be used for this purpose (or a combination of the two). These oils burn their eyes and scent glands, destroying them. Pump spray the air all about you to drive them off.
• take oil of oregano under the tongue and/or squirt into the mouth, as much as possible.

Bell's palsy

This condition, which afflicts tens of thousands of Americans yearly, is caused by paralysis of a nerve that controls the muscles of the face. The muscles simply refuse to work, because the nerves supplying them have become disabled. It is caused by a virus, which attacks the nerve, causing inflammation and swelling, disrupting the function of the nerve. Ultimately, it is the swelling that causes the problem, because this places great pressure on the nerve, blocking the flow of nerve impulses.

The involved nerve controls the strength of the muscles of the face, but when it is infected, this function fails. This explains the typical symptoms of Bell's palsy. Each side of the face has one of these nerves, and, since only one side of the facial nerve is infected, only one side is damaged. Bell's palsy symptoms include inability to wrinkle the brow, inability to close the eyelids (the eye stays open), inability to make a voluntary facial expression (like a smile), numbness of the face and lips, pain behind the ear, and excessive tearing. Aggressive treatment of this condition is necessary, because unless the swelling is reduced and the virus killed, permanent damage is likely.

Bell's palsy combat kit
• oil of lavender — rub under nose or on inside of nostrils. Rub on face and forehead.
• oil of oregano (use of the SuperStrength may be necessary) —

rub over the check, facial bones, and behind the ear on the affected side. Take two or more drops under the tongue several times daily until the problem is solved.

• oil of rosemary — 2 drops under the tongue 5 times daily. Take also 10 drops in juice or water twice daily.
• pantothenic acid — take 500 mg (as capsules) every three hours.
• vitamin A eye drops — for dry or exposed eyes
• BromaZyme — take 2 or 3 capsules three times daily on an empty stomach.

Bite wounds

At some point fully half of all North Americans will be bitten by some type of animal or another person. Such wounds may induce great physical and emotional trauma but also readily become infected. Certain infections are life threatening, notably tetanus and rabies. However, the latter can be prevented if the bite is treated immediately with antiseptic compounds and/or immunizations.

According to Presutti, writing in *Post Graduate Medicine,* dog bites are the most common type, accounting for as many as 2,000,000 bites per year. With their powerful jaws dogs can greatly traumatize the tissues, because they are capable of exerting hundreds of pounds of pressure. Thus, their bites may puncture the skin but may also bruise or traumatize deeply, even to the bone. Cat and human bites also readily become infected.

Bite combat kit
• oil of oregano — apply liberally to wound as often as necessary and take 2 drops under the tongue twice daily.
• oil of lavender — apply to wound liberally as often as necessary.
• Oil of Bay Berry — apply to wound; dramatic for inducing healing and for softening skin (i.e. preventing scarring).
• vitamin E (internally and externally to prevent scarring).
• bromelain (uncoated) — take 3 or more capsules twice daily on an empty stomach.

Bladder infection

Bladder infections are a nightmare no matter what the circumstance. Known medically as cystitis, these infections cause an enormous degree of disability. Yet, natural remedies are proven to minimize, perhaps cure, this condition.

The majority of infections are caused by bacteria, E. coli being the most notorious. Yeasts are also a common cause, especially in individuals who have taken repeated doses of antibiotics. One of the greatest risk factors for recurrent bladder infections is mechanical invasion of the bladder. Thus, individuals who have had prolonged surgeries resulting in catheter placement and/or anyone who has had scopes inserted in the bladder or penis has a high risk for infection, particularly by yeasts. If the individual has been previously catheterized and is suffering from recurrent kidney or bladder infections, it is virtually assured that yeast infection is the cause.

Bladder infection combat kit
• oil of fennel (a great urinary flushing agent) — take 5 to 10 drops twice daily.
• oil of oregano — take a few drops under the tongue three times daily and 5 to 10 drops in juice or water twice daily.
• wild oregano capsules (Oregamax caps) — take 3 capsules three times daily.
• cranberry capsules — take several capsules or as directed, three or four times daily.
• red grape powder (Resvitanol) — take 4 to 6 capsules three times daily (or 1 teaspoon three or four times daily).

Foods that help
• Welch's Grape Juice
• cranberry juice concentrate or pure unsweetened cranberry juice
• raw honey (for bacterial infections only; sugar feeds yeast)
• watermelon (natural urine and bacteria flushing agent)

Things to avoid
• citrus juice
• caffeine, coffee, tea, and iced tea
• sugar and chocolate

Bleeding Gums

Bleeding gums are a warning sign of nutritional deficiency, indicating a lack of vitamin C and/or bioflavonoids. In the extreme bleeding gums represent an early sign of scurvy.

When the gums break down, they are readily invaded by germs. The germs must be destroyed for the gums to heal and the bleeding to be stopped. Antiseptic herbs, such as cloves, bay, oregano, and tea tree, especially their oils, are effective and safe for reversing this condition.

Bleeding gums combat kit
• oil of oregano — rub on gums, a.m. and p.m; also, use on toothbrush.
• Flavin-C — take 4 to 8 capsules daily.
• folic acid – take 5 mg daily.
• Oregamax capsules (also a source of gum/teeth nourishing trace minerals such as calcium, zinc, and magnesium) — take 2 or 3 capsules twice daily.
• Resvitanol —take 1 t. or 4 to 6 capsules daily.

Things to avoid
• white sugar (causes the degeneration of the bone that sets the teeth, the enamel, and the gums)
• soda pop (phosphoric acid and sugar destroy enamel and damage bone)

Bleeding wounds

What can be done if an individual is bleeding to death? Certainly, the person must be rushed to the hospital. Yet, the more common disaster is minor-moderate bleeding, which is treatable.

Only a few natural substances act as clotting agents, that is they halt bleeding. When applied topically, these agents stop bleeding as well as speed the healing of wounds. These substances include garlic, onion, and essential oils. Phenol rich oils are the best clotting agents. Simply drip the oils on the wound. You may need to apply slight pressure (with a clean cotton ball or bandage). When applied to the skin, oil of oregano is an aggressive clotting agent.

Repeat as needed until bleeding halts. The effects are virtually miraculous. For shaving cuts it is a lifesaver.

Bleeding wounds combat kit
• oil of oregano (SuperStrength is best) — add directly to the wound/cut; if bleeding fails to stop immediately, apply firm (but not excessive) pressure until it stops.
• oil of lavender — apply to wound and on surrounding skin.
• Flavin-C — to heal any wound and help minimize bleeding take 2 to 3 capsules twice daily. For severe bleeding take 2 or more capsules every half hour or every hour.
• red grape powder (Resvitanol) — a tremendously valuable circulatory aid and clotting normalizing agent. Take 2 to 4 capsules every few hours. For more severe problems take 6 capsules several times daily or a teaspoonful several times daily. The powder, which possesses astringent properties, may also be dusted on the wound.
Note: the best method (outside of surgical intervention) for stopping bleeding from a gushing wound is heavy pressure by applying, preferably, sterile gauze or a clean cloth. Pressure plus essential oils is highly effective.

Blood clots
Blood clots are of two types; the type that is within the surface tissues, that is in the veins just under the skin, or the deep type, which cannot be felt or seen and which is in the deep veins or organs of the body. Both of these are medical emergencies, although medical treatment for the superficial type is often minimal.

Blood clot combat kit
• oil of oregano — rub over involved area. Take 2 drops under the tongue several times daily.
• bromelain (BromaZyme) — take 4 capsules 4 to 6 times daily, preferably on an empty stomach.
• onion juice — if the clot is in the leg or arm, soak a cloth in onion juice and wrap around involved area. Drink a cup of the juice daily.
• oil of lavender — gently rub over involved area. Take also two drops under the tongue twice daily.

Foods that help
- sardines, salmon, albacore tuna, mackerel, and herring
- onions and garlic (raw)
- papaya and its seeds
- raw fresh pineapple

Boils

There are two types of boils: carbuncles and furuncles. The distinction is that carbuncles are infections within the sebaceous glands of the skin, while furuncles are infections within the hair follicles. The latter condition commonly occurs in men with heavy beards, who shave frequently. Shaving traumatizes the delicate facial skin. This allows germs to gain entry to the hair follicles, in which they multiply.

Black males are particularly susceptible to developing extensive boils, largely due to ingrown hairs on the face and other regions. These boils often occur in large numbers on the cheeks and/or neck and are quite disfiguring.

Most furuncles and carbuncles are caused by staph and/or strep infections. Infection by yeasts may be a contributing factor.

While boils are often painful and/or disfiguring, they are not regarded as a serious condition. However, if left untreated, they may persist for weeks or months. Systemic antibiotic therapy usually fails to eradicate them. The drugs can't penetrate the site of the infection. Plus, the infections are often caused by antibiotic-resistant microbes, staph and strep being the most notorious of these. People who live in close quarters, such as athletic teams or hospitalized patients, may suffer from outbreaks of staphylococcal boils.

Boil combat kit
- oil of oregano — apply to the involved sites; take also 5 to 10 drops internally daily.
- Oil of Bay Berry — apply to involved areas.
- oil of myrtle — apply to involved areas.
- vitamin E (as mixed tocopherols) — take 800 to 1200 I.U.
- bromelain — take 2 capsules twice daily on an empty stomach.

• primrose or borage oil — take 4 capsules twice daily.

Foods that help
• papaya plus the seeds and/or dried papaya spears
• sunflower seeds, raw
• fatty fish of all types

Things to avoid
• caffeine, coffee, chocolate, tea, iced tea
• deep fried foods

Bone infection (osetomyelitis)

This infection usually occurs as a consequence of trauma or surgery. It is caused by bacteria, which lodge into the bone, eating away at it. Most commonly, it develops in leg bones. Smokers and diabetics are at the highest risk.

The hallmark for this disastrous illness is an open wound or a hole in the skin, which drains pus or other secretions. This is called a draining sinus, and the opening may be large or relatively small. This is apparently the body's way of eliminating the poisons, which are pent up within the bone. The usual culprit is staph, although Pseudomonas, a very obnoxious and difficult to kill microbe, may also cause it. Bone infection may develop without trauma or surgery. No one is sure how this happens, but this certainly signifies that the immune system is dysfunctional: the bones are normally sterile.

Bone infections nearly always result when compound fractures develop in disaster circumstances. This is because there is no means to keep the tissues sterile.

Bone infection combat kit
• culture the site and take appropriate antibiotics (if available).
• oil of oregano SuperStrength — take internally and put on or into the wound.
• oil of lavender — rub over wound site and/or put in wound.
• oil of bay leaf — take 10 to 20 drops twice daily.
• wild oregano herb (Oregamax capsules) — take 3 or more

capsules twice daily.
• bromelain (use only the uncoated assayed variety, i.e. BromaZyme) — take 3 or more capsules three times daily on an empty stomach.

Bronchitis

As described in *Patient Care* magazine, January, 1996, medical doctors claim that they don't know the cause of bronchitis. What's more, they state that antibiotics are virtually useless for curing it. *Taber's Medical Dictionary* defines bronchitis as "inflammation in the bronchial tubes." Something has to be causing the inflammation, and that something is usually infection. Food allergies are a secondary but important cause. Dissolving the inflammation is certainly helpful in resolving this condition. However, if the bronchial tubes are infected, the offending germ must be destroyed in order for resolution to occur.

Patients are commonly bombarded with multiple doses of antibiotics in attempt to cure the disease. However, according to current research viruses are the primary cause of bronchitis, not bacteria. Plus, if the condition is caused by food allergies, antibiotics aggravate it. Even if bacteria are involved, they are usually immune to antibiotics. Thus, the approach to treatment must be totally different than the current method. This illustrates the value of using natural antiseptics and antiinflammatory agents, both of which combat the causes of this condition.

Bronchitis combat kit
• oil of oregano — take 2 drops under the tongue, as often as necessary. Take also 5 drops three times daily in juice or water.
• wild oregano capsules (Oregamax) — take 3 capsules three times daily.
• oil of rosemary (for opening up lung passages) — rub on chest and take 5 to 10 drops twice daily.
• oil of cilantro/coriander — take 5 to 10 drops twice daily.
• Essence of Orange Blossom (or White Coffee) or Essence of Rose 2Petals — add 2 tablespoons of either one to hot water as a

tea; drink as often as needed.
• Flavin-C — take 3 capsules three times daily.
• oil of lavender — rub on chest and under nose; take 2 drops under the tongue twice daily (for this purpose use only the edible oil of lavender emulsified in extra virgin olive oil).

Foods that help
• horseradish, freshly grated if possible
• raw onion and garlic
• onion/garlic/meat broths
• raw honey

Things to avoid
• milk products, especially butter and cheese
• chocolate
• wheat and rye

Bruises
This condition results from trauma which is sufficient enough to break blood vessels. The broken blood vessels allow the leakage of blood into the tissues, leading to the reddish-brown or purplish color of the bruise. In some individuals bruises develop without obvious trauma. This is an early sign of scurvy and represents a significant deficiency of vitamin C and bioflavonoids. It may also tell of fungal infection in the gut. The fungi crowd out the good bacteria, such as Lactobacillus, which are responsible for synthesizing a special clotting factor: vitamin K. Killing the yeasts allows the return of the good bacteria, thus helping to normalize vitamin K synthesis.

Bruise Combat Kit
• oil of oregano — apply topically to dissipate the bruises (it works for this rather dramatically).
• Flavin-C — take 3 capsules three times daily.
• oil of rosemary (rich in flavonoids) — take 5 to 10 drops twice daily.

• WildPower Tea — drink one or two cups of this brew daily.
• oil of myrtle (rich in flavonoids) — take 2 to 5 drops twice daily and rub on the involved region.

Foods that help
• tangerines and grapefruit (and their juices, eat the inner rind)
• watercress, arugula, and spinach
• frozen unpasteurized orange juice (this is usually made from ripe oranges, which are higher in vitamin C than the so-called fresh ones)
• rose hip tea or, preferably, Essence of Rose Petal tea

Burns

Burns are among the most traumatic of all injuries, both physically and mentally. If a burn covers a small surface area, like a bit of the finger, the trauma is tolerable. However, if it covers large areas, like a part of the arm or torso, the body may suffer from severe stress—perhaps shock. If the burn is caused by a noxious chemical, such as lye or bleach, the shock is due to severe trauma to the tissues but also the absorption of the chemical through the skin and/or inhalation. The point is burns are not just painful, blistered skin; they impact the entire body. Any burn covering more than an inch is highly traumatic to the body. The pain alone is enough to create shock in certain individuals.

Burn combat kit
• oil of oregano — apply to the region liberally, and take a few drops under the tongue as often as necessary.
• Oil of Bay Berry — apply to region as needed.
• oil of lavender — apply to region as needed.
• aloe vera — apply to region (usually after applying essential oils)
• bromelain — for large scale burns to reduce swelling and trauma, take 3 capsules several times daily on an empty stomach.
• raw honey — apply to any burn either by itself or after applying essential oils.

Things to avoid
• bandages that stick to the skin. It is preferable to leave the wound open.

Canker sores

These are usually induced by food intolerance, that is food allergy. Sensitivity to chemicals in the foods, as well as prescription and/or non-prescription drugs, is another cause. Certain researchers believe that infection plays a role in canker sores and that strep or perhaps viruses are partly to blame. However, food allergy is the number one provoking factor. British researchers found that wheat was the major canker sore inducing food. Other allergenic foods include rye, corn, milk products, beans, citrus fruit, shrimp, peanuts, and chocolate.

Canker sore combat kit
• oil of oregano — apply to involved region and take 2 drops under the tongue twice daily.
• oil of rosemary — apply to involved region and take a few drops twice daily in juice or water.
• Royal Kick — take 3 capsules twice daily.
• oil of sage (soothing; anti-pain) — apply a few drops on involved region.
• folic acid — take 3 or more mg twice daily.

Things to avoid
• all grains, especially wheat (flour products are the #1 offender)
• milk products, especially butter
• citrus fruit and juices
• nuts, beans, and legumes

Carbon monoxide poisoning

This is primarily a problem of smoke inhalation. With a hidden carbon monoxide leak, such as might occur from a leaky furnace, by the time it is noticed it is usually too late to apply a natural remedy. I experienced a near fatal carbon monoxide event. While on a fishing trip in the remote wilderness, our group stayed in a rudimentary cabin. One of the members was an adolescent, a rather unpredictable individual. Tired of the endless barrage of mosquitoes, he thought that by plugging up the outside vent to the heater he would block them from entering. Blocked it was, that is the carbon monoxide. Asphixiated during the night we awoke well after fishing time in a stupor, tired and incoherent. Fortunately, the windows were cracked, or it is likely that everyone in our party would have died. At least it would have happened amongst Nature.

This incident was a more rare means for being poisoned. Tens of thousands of Americans develop carbon monoxide poisoning in ways that are not usually fatal but still devastate health. For instance, boaters are at high risk. This is particularly true of boats with enclosed cabins. Fishermen who troll using gas motors are at risk. Smoke inhalation from fires is a major cause of carbon monoxide toxicity. Perhaps the greatest cause is a type of chronic contamination. This is usually from oil furnaces and gas stoves, which seep carbon monoxide into homes, causing chronic illness. This is not a rare disease, and as many as 100,000 Americans suffer some degree of carbon monoxide poisoning every year.

The medical treatment of carbon monoxide exposure is oxygen, the ideal form being an oxygen chamber. Such facilities are unavailable in most hospitals and will be inaccessible in the event of major crises. Symptoms of carbon monoxide poisoning include:
- headache (one of the earliest signs and may be severe)
- fatigue
- weakness
- incoherence
- dizziness
- nausea or upset stomach
- apathy
- muscular exhaustion
- cherry red complexion

Note: the above symptoms are often mistaken for the flu.

Carbon monoxide detoxification kit

- oil of rosemary — take 5 drops under the tongue several times daily plus 10 drops in juice or water twice daily.
- Juice of Rosemary — drink an ounce several times daily.
- Juice of Oregano — drink an ounce several times daily.
- oil of sage — take 10 drops twice daily.
- beta carotene — take 50,000 I.U. of natural source beta carotene daily.
- vitamin E as mixed tocopherols — take 400 I.U. several times daily until condition resolves.
- selenium (organic) — take 250 mg three times daily.

Foods that help

- tomato paste mixed with olive oil
- pumpkin and butternut squash
- red radishes (and their tops if possible; make radish juice from the tops and drink a cup daily)

Things to avoid

- any exposure to smoke or fumes; even a tiny amount can be disabling; also, avoid nitrated/processed meats.

Chapped lips

This annoying condition is rarely ameliorated with lip balms alone. Actually, this problem may be caused by nutritional deficiencies. Deficiencies of essential fatty acids, folic acid, riboflavin, and vitamin A may all play a role. To treat this condition take a multiple vitamin containing vitamins A, folic acid, riboflavin, and vitamin C. Take also essential fatty acids, for instance, primrose or flax oil. Use a natural herbal based lip balm. Take additional folic acid, 5 mg daily. Other invaluable substances include healing essential oils such as oils of bay berry, myrtle, and lavender.

Chickenpox

This is one of the most contagious of all diseases. It is caused by a virus: the Herpes virus. The chickenpox (herpes) virus usually attacks children, who have no immunity to it. If an outbreak occurs, fully 80% of all non-immune sensitized individuals exposed to it will become infected, including adults. However, it usually strikes children ages 4 to 8 years. Infants are occasionally infected, and it can be quite serious in this age group. Ironically, chickenpox in adults is usually more severe than in children; life-threatening pneumonia is often a consequence. Adults exposed to the virus while taking steroid therapy are at the highest risk for severe infections, since cortisone of all types may provoke the infection and drive it deep into the tissues. If the infection is severe enough, brain damage can occur (usually in children/infants).

Chickenpox combat kit for children
• oil of oregano — take 1 drop under the tongue or in juice or water every three hours. Rub on chest, thighs, buttocks, and/or soles of feet.
• oil of lavender — rub on chest liberally as well as the soles of the feet; also, rub vigorously on the buttocks. Do this at least twice daily.
• Flavin-C — take 2 capsules three times daily.
• Oregamax capsules — take 2 capsules three times daily.
• crude raw honey — take a tablespoon three times daily.

Chickenpox combat kit for adults
• oil of oregano — take 2 drops under the tongue every hour until condition improves; then 2 drops every few hours.
• Oregamax capsules — take 3 capsules three times daily.
• Flavin-C — take 3 or more capsules three times daily.
• Royal Kick — take 3 or more capsules twice daily.

Things to avoid
• soda pop and sugar
• chocolate: absolutely none of any kind

Chlorine gas/liquid poisoning

Chlorine is a highly noxious substance which is extremely corrosive to human tissues. Millions of tons of chlorine gas and liquid chlorine are transported by rail car and truck yearly. Other millions of tons are stored in factories and depots virtually everywhere. Chlorine gas/liquid spills are relatively common events in the United States, afflicting thousands of individuals every year. The unfortunate people who live near factories, as well as industrial workers, are the usual victims.

Note: a chlorine spill and resultant gas cloud are extremely dangerous. Be aggressive in taking antioxidants such as wild oil of oregano, edible oil of rosemary, oil of cumin, oil of wild sage, and selenium; this may save your lungs and perhaps your life.

Chlorine exposure combat kit

* gas mask and protective clothing
* oil of cumin — take 10 drops internally every hour and a few drops under the tongue frequently, about every 15 minutes.
* oil of rosemary — take 10 drops internally every hour and a few drops under the tongue every few minutes.
* oil of oregano — take 2 drops under the tongue every few minutes to prevent respiratory collapse.
* organic selenium — take 200 mcg every six/eight hours. Use this dosage only for emergencies.
* Flavin-C — take 2 capsules every hour.
* oil of sage (a powerful antioxidant and lung protector) — take 2 drops under the tongue every half hour.
* Juice of Sage — drink two or more ounces daily until the exposure ends.
* Juice of Rosemary — drink an entire bottle daily until the exposure ends.
* Resvitanol — take 2 or 3 capsules every hour.
* chlorella — take as much of this as possible.

Cholera

This is a highly contagious intestinal infection caused by the obnoxious pathogen, *Vibrio cholerae.* Currently, cholera is responsible for hundreds of thousands of deaths yearly, mostly in poor countries. Yet, outbreaks could occur anywhere. This is because cholera is a water borne disease, and the responsible germ could contaminate any water system.

A bout of cholera could probably kill even Hercules, in other words, no one is immune. The germ viciously attacks the intestines, particularly the small bowel. It causes bile stained profuse watery diarrhea, plus vomiting (which is usually violent) and severe intestinal cramps. Nothing seemingly can stop the diarrhea. The stools have what is known as a "rice in water" appearance. Yet, if the organism is killed, the diarrhea will stop. Unstopped, the individual usually dies from dehydration.

The infection notoriously fails to respond to even the most heroic medical efforts, thus illustrating the importance of natural therapies. A variety of natural substances have been shown to halt diarrhea and destroy noxious germs. These remedies include oil of oregano, oil of cumin, oil of cinnamon, raw honey, garlic, and natural (normal) flora.

It was Eli Metnickoff, the man who popularized yogurt, who did the cholera challenge. After taking large amounts of yogurt over a period of time, he drank a dose of cholera. He failed to contract the disease. Thus, his system was apparently protected by the natural Lactobacillus which he had consumed via the yogurt.

There are no effective drugs or vaccines for this condition. Thus, the individual must depend upon natural cures. If you contract cholera, don't eat anything, in other words, rest the gut. Seek medical attention. Sip on clear fluids, and use the natural remedies described herein. Be aggressive with these remedies: your life may depend upon it.

Cholera Combat Kit

• crude raw honey — take large amounts, like a quarter cup three times daily. Continue the honey therapy for at least 3 days.
• oil of oregano (SuperStrength is best) — take a few drops under the tongue repeatedly until the diarrhea slows down or halts.
• oil of cumin — take 5 to 10 drops internally several times daily.
• Lactobacillus — if this can be held down, take several capsules throughout the day.
• papaya seeds — if this can be held down, pulverize and add to

water. Or, take papain capsules, i.e. papaya enzymes (BromaZyme).
• raw garlic — this is irritating to the gut but may be the only remedy available. Thoroughly chew cloves and eat repeatedly.

Foods that help
• garlic/onion broth
• vinegar
• raw honey
• orange blossom tea
• rose petal essence

Other ideals: rest the gut as much as possible; use raw honey/vinegar, broths, and teas for fluid replenishment.

Cold exposure (Coldness of the body, hands, feet, etc.)
Exposure to cold weather and the resulting cold body temperature are a great concern in human crisis. Could significant crises afflict this country so that common conveniences, such as heating and shelter, are unavailable? This happened in 1998 during the great ice storms in the upper northeastern United States and Canada. It could possibly happen as a result of the Y2K dilemma, because the power grids are computer controlled. What will individuals do—how will they behave—if they are unable to keep warm, that is if the common conveniences of everyday life are disrupted? Perhaps some individuals might even harm others to gain their security.

Cold body temperature protection/combat kit
• oil of oregano — take 2 to 4 drops under the tongue three times daily. Rub on face and hands a few moments before going outside.
• cayenne pepper — add to food; sprinkle on socks to prevent frostbite.
• garlic supplements (or cloves) — eat one raw clove daily.
• onions, raw — eat one bulb daily.
• Oregamax capsules (contains wild oregano, garlic, and onion) — take 2 or more capsules twice daily.
• kelp — take 4 capsules (about 1000 mg) of arsenic free kelp daily.
• oil of sage (highly warming) — if possible, make oil of sage tea

by adding several drops to hot water. Also, take oil of sage, 5 to 10 drops daily.
• oil of cilantro plus coriander (highly warming) — take 5 to 10 drops twice daily.

Foods that protect
• sardines, salmon, albacore tuna, mackerel
• crude extra virgin olive oil
• salted roasted nuts
• fresh beef (as steaks, chops, roasts, stews, broth — marrow soup is particularly nourishing, the fattier it is the better it is for cold protection)

Cold sores

Cold sores are caused by a virus, specifically the Herpes virus type I. This virus apparently resides in the majority of Americans, parasitizing the cells of the nervous system. Usually, it remains dormant, hiding deep within the nerve tissues. However, when the individual is subjected to extreme stress or is taking certain medications, such as cortisone or chemotherapy, the virus ruptures through the nerves and into the skin. This results in extensive inflammation and, thus, severe pain.

Cold sore combat kit
• oil of oregano — apply immediately and repeatedly directly to the lesion when you feel the tingle. Take 2 or more drops under the tongue several times daily or until the lesion clears.
• lysine — (more of a preventive than a cure)
• Royal Kick premium royal jelly (to combat stress and reverse adrenal weakness) — take 2 capsules every few hours.
• Oregamax — take 2 capsules every few hours.
• oil of sage — apply directly to the lesion repeatedly.

Foods that help
• anything rich in all eight essential amino acids, that is beef, chicken, fish, eggs, and milk products
• fatty fish such as sardines, salmon, albacore tuna, and mackerel
• fresh whole milk mixed with honey

Things to avoid
- chocolate (like the plague)
- peanuts and peanut butter
- refined vegetable oils and deep fried foods

Colds

This condition may be caused by viruses. The term "'may"
will surprise certain individuals, because the medical profession
has taught that colds are always caused by viruses. However, there
is another insidious cause: mold. Allergic intolerance to mold or
infection by yeasts/molds may mimic a viral cold.

     Cold viruses attack primarily the nasal passages, sinuses,
and throat, that is the upper respiratory tract. They parasitize the
cells in these regions. They also attack the lymph glands, notably
the tonsils, adenoids, and lymph nodules. Bombard them where
they live with essential oils and other remedies aimed directly at the
site of infection.

Cold combat kit
- oil of oregano — a powerful, effective remedy; take two drops
under the tongue several times per day. For severe colds take two
drops under the tongue every hour, and rub around the sinus region.
Because of its immense anti-fungal action, this is an outright cure
for the common cold.
- raw honey plus vinegar — use this often as a food and tonic until
the cold dissipates.
- Oregamax capsules — take 3 capsules three or more times daily.
- Flavin-C — take 2 or more capsules every hour.
- oil of cilantro/coriander — take 5 to 10 drops several times daily.

Foods that help
- fresh juices, especially vitamin C-rich ones like tangerine,
papaya, grapefruit, and strawberry juice
- meat or poultry broth with onion and garlic
- canned tomato juice; drink two quarts daily.

Things to avoid
- white sugar and/or chocolate; these are disastrous foods to
consume during a cold
- milk products

Colic

This term is a bit of a misnomer, because it seems like it defines a colon problem. Yet, the term is used for any type of spasm in the abdomen. Today, it applies almost exclusively to children.

Childhood colic is usually a minor problem. The objective is to settle the stomach or intestines so the child (and parents) can rest. Essential oils are the optimal agent for this purpose. They possess considerable powers to relax the stomach and intestines, quickly reversing spasticity and/or pain. There is no medical treatment for baby colic, all the more reason to utilize natural cures.

Colic combat kit
• oil of lavender — rub on the soles of the feet, over abdomen, and on buttocks.
• oil of oregano — rub on soles of feet and over abdomen.
• Juice of Oregano — give a small amount, like a tablespoonful, to halt colic.
• Essence of Orange Blossom — gentle, but effective; give a teaspoon or more in goat milk, formula, or juice.
• oil of fennel — used since antiquity, a famous English remedy; two or three drops daily should be sufficient.
• oil of ginger — one or two drops of the edible type daily

Things to avoid
• caffeine, chocolate, sugar, coffee, and cow's milk

Colitis attacks

This category covers a wide range of bowel disorders, which may collectively be grouped under this heading. These disorders include irritable bowel syndrome, spastic colon, Crohn's disease, and ulcerative colitis.

These conditions are plagues of modern civilization. They are directly due to erroneous diet. Food allergies and infection also play an important role. Emotional distress is another major cause of colonic disorders. Stress, despair, and worry, as well as the emotion of guilt, all are largely to blame. Why these emotions specifically attack the bowel is unknown.

The colon illnesses are manifested by severe toxicity

affecting the entire digestive tract, although the colon suffers the brunt of the damage. Symptoms include diarrhea as well as constipation, cramps, spasticity, mucousy stools, bleeding in the stools, hemorrhoids, nausea, and bloating. Untreated, it may lead to infections throughout the body and, ultimately, colon cancer.

Colitis combat kit
• oil of oregano — take 2 drops under the tongue several times daily. Plus, take Oreganol gelcaps, two caps twice daily.
• Oregamax capsules — take 2 or more capsules three times daily.
• oil of sage (a relaxant to the gut and aids the coping mechanism—the adrenals) — take 5 drops twice daily in hot water.
• oil of wild myrtle in extra virgin olive oil (a tremendous aid to spasticity) 5 or more drops twice daily
• oil of rosemary (blocks spasticity and nourishes the gut wall) — take 5 to 10 drops twice daily in juice or water.
• oil of fennel or oil of ginger (highly important for normalizing the gut) — take 3 to 5 drops twice daily.

Things to avoid
• all sources of caffeine
• refined sugar and corn syrup
• wheat and flour products of all types
• beans and legumes
• milk products of all types, especially milk, ice cream, and butter

Concussion
One of the most common human injuries, concussion is especially prevalent in children. It is caused by direct trauma to the skull. In mild cases no damage is done. However, with extreme injury temporary or permanent brain damage may occur. This may be manifested by insomnia, headaches, amnesia, and even permanent neurological deficit.

Concussion combat kit
• oil of lavender — rub all over face and head, especially under the nose. Rub on soles of feet. Do this repeatedly until an

improvement in consciousness is noted.
• oil of oregano — rub on chest and face; take 2 drops under the tongue several times daily until condition improves.
• oil of bay leaf — rub on face and chest several times daily.
• Flavin-C — take 2 capsules every hour (especially valuable to prevent internal bleeding).
• Essence of Orange Blossom — gently activates and stimulates brain function; eases stress; add 2 tablespoons to hot water and sip. Repeat as needed.
• wild St. John's wort — take 2 capsules twice daily.

Things to avoid
• loud noises and bright light; Note: keep the individual in a dark quiet room until help arrives.

Conjunctivitis

Hurricane Georges struck the American South like a hydrogen bomb. It blasted through the U. S. Virgin Islands in September, 1998, destroying thousands of homes and displacing thousands. One of the consequences was the spread of infection, and conjunctivitis was top on the list. Pink eye incidence was 30 times higher than normal as a result of the hurricane.

Conjunctivitis is defined as inflammation or irritation of the eye membranes that cover the whites of the eyes and also the membranes of the inner eyelid. A red inflamed eye is the same as conjunctivitis. It is commonly caused by infection, particularly bacteria and viruses. Thus, most cases of red eye signal infection. Red eye can also be caused when foreign objects become trapped in the membranes of the eyes such as particles of dust, sand, metal, or wood. Even so, when such particles are trapped for prolonged periods, infection often develops. If there is a discharge that tends to form a crust, especially if foul smelling, infection of the eye or inner eyelid is assured. Red irritated eyes which itch usually signals allergic reactions. Exposure to toxic chemicals, especially if they are airborne, may be a major cause of red or inflamed eyes. Signs and symptoms of acute bacterial conjunctivitis include:

- burning
- automatic tearing
- irritation
- yellowish, yellow-green, or pus filled discharge
- swelling of the eyelids

Viral infections of the eyes are potentially a catastrophic dilemma. This is because viruses spread easily, and viral conjunctivitis may become epidemic, especially in medical facilities or in institutions housing large numbers of people. Careful hand washing reduces the risk of transmission. Typical symptoms include red eyes, watery discharge, swelling of the eyelids, and sensation of something in the eye. Such infections are usually contagious for at least one week.

Viral eye infections may be caused by herpes, and this can become dangerous. Never use cortisone creams in the event of viral/herpetic eye infections, as this may cause the virus to spread, permanently damaging and scarring the eye.

Conjunctivitis combat kit
- oil of oregano — take 2 drops under the tongue twice daily. Rub a small amount on cheeks under the eye (be sure to avoid any direct contact with eyeball. Use only edible oil of wild oregano emulsified in extra virgin olive oil). Remember, it travels.
- oil of wild lavender — rub on forehead and cheeks around eyes (but not in eyes).
- vitamin A eye drops — add one drop in involved eye twice daily.
- Flavin-C (as a source of crude natural vitamin C and bioflavonoids) — take 3 capsules twice daily.

Constipation
Constipation is a disease only of modern civilization. In this condition the colon fails to eliminate wastes efficiently. Symptoms include abdominal pain, bloating, gas, headaches, bad breath, and fatigue. When movements finally occur, the stool is usually hard and dark. A good definition is having less than a bowel movement per day. Extreme constipation is having less than a bowel movement per week.

It has been proposed that a lack of dietary fiber is the primary cause of constipation. Yet, this is only one factor. Food allergy, as well as chronic infection, are other major causes. Dehydration is another important factor. Perhaps the most neglected issue is the fact that constipation may be a key sign of intestinal infection. Parasitic infection is a major cause of constipation. The bulk of the parasites itself may plug up the bowel, making it difficult to have a movement. Yeast infections can also cause chronic constipation.

There has been a gross overemphasis upon using harsh laxatives, whether chemical or herbal, in attempt to cure constipation. The problem is that the bowel becomes damaged from the aggressive powers of many laxatives, and, as soon as these agents are halted, the constipation returns. If you use herbal laxatives, take them for a short period for purposes of detoxification, not every day.

Constipation combat kit
- oil of oregano — take 2 drops twice daily in juice or water.
- Oregamax — take 3 capsules two or three times daily.
- red grape powder (Resvitanol) — take 4 capsules three times daily (or take a heaping teaspoonful twice daily).
- Nutri-Sense — take 3 heaping tablespoons twice daily in juice or water.
- BromaZyme (to stimulate digestion) — take 2-3 capsules with meals.
- PureKelp (helps stimulate/enhance colonic muscle function) — take 4 capsules daily.

Foods that help
- Nutri-Sense drink/food mix or ground flax
- papaya plus the seeds
- wild rice (and/or rice bran)
- wild rosemary (or Hercules Strength capsules)
- carob molasses — a highly effective gentle agent, non-habit forming bowel aid. Add this to the Nutri-Sense for a natural means for balancing colon function. It works!

Note: be sure to increase fluid intake and drink at least 6 large glasses of water daily.

Things to avoid
- refined sugar
- anything made with white flour and/or hydrogenated oils

Cough

A cough may be a rather mild problem. However, it may also become a disability. A persistent cough is one of the most disabling of all symptoms. It is tiring as well as damaging, both to the lungs and nerves. Persistent deep coughs may also damage internal organs, particularly the esophagus and/or stomach.

A cough is a sign that lung function is compromised. This is usually due to an infection, although chemical poisoning as well as allergic sensitivity may provoke it. Persistent cough with no obvious cause may also warn of cancer. However, usually, it signals chronic infection by bacteria, fungi, viruses, or parasites. Currently, mold/yeast infection of the lungs represents perhaps the number one cause of chronic cough.

Cough combat kit
- oil of oregano — take 2 or more drops under the tongue three or more times daily. Also, rub on chest, around sinuses, and under nose.
- oil of myrtle — rub on chest; take 2 to 5 drops twice daily.
- black seed extract (Black seed-plus or Herb-Sorb) — 2 capsules three times daily.
- Oil of Bay Berry — rub on chest and face; take 2 to 5 drops twice daily.
- oil of lavender — rub on face and chest as well as soles of the feet.
- Oregamax capsules — take 3 capsules twice daily.
- Essence of Rose Petals (highly soothing and warming) — add 2 tablespoons to hot water and drink as a tea as often as desired. The Essence of Orange Blossoms may be taken for the same usage.
- kelp (arsenic-free) — take 4 or more capsules daily.
- oil of sage — take 5 drops twice daily in hot water.

Foods that help
- wild sage herb (for making tea)
- iodine-rich foods such as sardines, salmon, halibut, etc.

Things to avoid
• milk products and chocolate
• wheat and other commercial grains (may provoke a type of mold sensitivity)

Cracks at the corners of the mouth

This painful condition is strictly caused by a vitamin deficiency. However, once the cracks develop, they may become invaded by germs, notably yeasts. The primary deficiency is riboflavin, although niacin and folic acid deficiencies may play secondary roles.

Vitamin/herbal cures
• royal jelly, naturally rich in riboflavin (500 mg capsules) — take 4-6 capsules daily. A crude completely unprocessed royal jelly is now available.
• riboflavin pills — take 50 to 100 milligrams per day.
• Oil of Bay Berry (soothing; stimulates healing) — apply topically.
• folic acid — take 5 mg daily.

Foods that help
• organic liver (the top source of riboflavin)
• whole eggs or egg powder (fair source of riboflavin)
• almonds or almond milk (good vegetable source of riboflavin)
• whole milk yogurt, whole milk, or milk powder (rich in riboflavin)
• watercress, spinach, and avocado
• wild rice and its broth

Croup

Croup is a respiratory crisis demanding immediate medical attention. It is a childhood condition manifested by odd breathing sounds or a cough resembling a bark. The child may also appear to be suffocating or wheezing. There is also loss of voice, difficult breathing, weakness, and rapid pulse. Croup may eventually be determined to be a type of diphtheria secondary to immunization reactions. Indeed, this illness, which may be provoked by immunizations, is often manifested by membrane formation in the throat, similar to that seen in diphtheria.

This is one of the most serious respiratory infections in children. Obviously, it requires medical support. Even so, natural remedies are of immense value. This is emphasized by *Taber's Medical Dictionary*, which states that "antibiotics (and other drugs) are of no...benefit." The following amounts apply to young children.

Croup combat kit
• oil of oregano — a drop under the tongue as often as tolerated, but no more than 10 drops daily. Rub additional oil on buttocks, chest, or soles of feet.
• oil of lavender — rub on face, chest, buttocks, and soles of feet.
• oil of myrtle — rub on face, chest, buttocks, and soles of feet.
• raw honey — give as many tablespoons as possible.
• kelp (arsenic free) — give as many capsules as possible (add to juice, etc.)

Foods that help
• clear vegetable or meat broths

Things to avoid
• chocolate and refined sugar
• junk food of any type

Cuts/lacerations
The average American's arsenal for combating injuries is pitiful. Usually, it consists of noxious smelling drug store items, which offer little versatility. After many years of usage few Americans have any confidence in these items, the results being just as disappointing as the odor. The familiar names include hydrogen peroxide, hexachlorphene, antibiotic ointments, rubbing alcohol, and iodine. These agents are poor choices in a crisis. What's more, they are incapable of aiding wound healing. In fact, they may impede it.

Natural substances greatly accelerate wound healing. What's more, many of these agents, notably oregano, bay leaf, bay berry, lavender, and rosemary oils, bee propolis, and raw honey, offer germ killing powers. Some of them, like oils of oregano, lavender, and bay berry, contribute significant pain killing properties.

Natural cures for cuts, lacerations, and other open wounds
• oil of oregano — apply as needed; take a drop or two under the tongue.
• raw honey — apply to wound, perhaps over the essential oils. Cover with bandage or leave uncovered.
• oil of lavender — apply to wound twice daily.
• Oil of Bay Berry (stimulates healing; soothing) — apply to wound or skin surrounding the region.
• red grape powder (a tremendous astringent) —take 6 or more capsules daily to aid in wound healing. Also, dust powder onto bandage and apply to wound.

Cyanide poisoning

Cyanide is perhaps the most poisonous of all chemicals. It is fatal in minute amounts. As little as a tenth of a gram can kill a grown man. Much has been disseminated regarding the toxic effects of consuming cyanide such as cyanide laced drugs. However, a far greater crisis is the disastrous consequences of inhaling it in the form of cyanide gas. This is what happened with the catastrophe of the Union Carbide plant in Bhopal, India; tens of thousands were killed and maimed as a result of the "accidental" release of cyanide gas. These gases are known chemically as hydrogen cyanide or hydrocyanic gas.

Thousands of tons of cyanide gas are transported by rail or truck in the United States every year. Plus, this lethal chemical is stored in chemical bins throughout the country. A release in a metropolitan area, as occurred in India, could kill thousands within minutes, while leaving other uncountable thousands permanently diseased. The disease resulting from cyanide gas exposure is gruesome; corrosion of the lungs, leading to permanent disability at best or a slow writhing brutal death due to suffocation.

Short of a gas mask and special protective clothing there is no means of fully guarding the body from exposure to cyanide gas. This is because cyanide compounds are rapidly absorbed throughout the tissues. After entering the lungs cyanide is quickly absorbed into the bloodstream. It also penetrates the skin, ultimately entering the blood and internal organs. There, it poisons the cells and organs thoroughly. It does so by halting the ability of the body to transport and use its most critical substance: oxygen. Without this life-giving substance, death rapidly ensues. However, while cyanide gas releases are rare, there is a more insidious cause for exposure: smoke inhalation. Modern building materials are cyanide-laced. Thus, many fire related deaths may in fact be due to the inhalation of cyanide gas, which is rapidly liberated during fires.

In the event of a massive release of cyanide gas the logistics of self-protection are overwhelming. Immediately don a mask, wear protective eye covering, and wear a plastic/resilient suit. If the latter is unavailable, wear a blast jacket, rain coat, or similar plasticized outerwear. Quickly mobilize away from the site of exposure or stay indoors, closing all doors and windows. Secure the building as air tight as possible. Take mega doses of the anti-toxic antioxidants. Signs and symptoms of cyanide poisoning include:

- burning of the eyes and respiratory passages
- shortness of breath and breathing distress
- petechiae (small hemorrhages on the skin)
- nausea and vomiting
- almond-like odor from the breath and skin
- severe convulsions and/or seizures
- cherry-red color of the skin
- faintness, dizziness, fainting, and/or collapse
- sweating

Note: acute cyanide poisoning usually results in death within 20 minutes and, thus, many of these symptoms are rarely seen. Cyanide poisons the body by irreversibly binding to red blood cells, preventing them from delivering oxygen to the tissues. Without oxygen, survival is impossible and death results precipitously. However, if protective gear is rapidly donned, sudden death may be averted. In this case the aforementioned symptoms may appear, because, no matter how well the individual is protected, a certain degree of exposure will occur. If any of these symptoms develop after toxic chemical exposure, seek medical attention immediately (if possible).

If exposure of any sort occurs, take huge amounts of the anti-toxic antioxidants. Take the doses repeatedly, in other words, hit it hard. This is the only chance of survival.

Cyanide exposure combat kit
- oil of oregano — take several drops under the tongue every few minutes.
- oil of rosemary — take several drops under the tongue every few minutes.
- oil of sage — take a few drops under the tongue every few minutes. Also, take 20 additional drops internally twice daily.
- Juice of Sage — drink an entire bottle or more.
- Juice of Oregano — drink an entire bottle or more.
- oil of cumin (for detoxification of the cyanide through the stool) — take 10 or more drops every hour until danger abates.
- red grape powder (Resvitanol) — take 4 to 6 capsules every hour (or one teaspoon each hour)
- organic selenium — take 200 mcg every hour (such a dosage is for emergencies only).
- Flavin-C — take 3 or more capsules every half hour or every hour.

Dehydration

This is a disorder not just of fluid loss, but it also represents the loss of critical elemental substances. Known as electrolytes, these substances include sodium, chloride, magnesium, and potassium. Usually, sodium and chloride are the main electrolytes lost in dehydration.

One of the main issues with dehydration is to know what are the signs and symptoms. This is because dehydration is one of the most under-diagnosed of all illnesses. The problem is no one suspects it, and, thus, it is frequently missed. This is particularly true of the elderly, who often fail to take care of themselves properly. In heat waves dehydration is a major cause of sickness and death in this population.

Hot weather is a major factor in causing dehydration, as is prolonged fever. The latter causes rapid fluid loss through both the skin and lungs. With fever, dehydration may develop in as little as a few hours. Diarrhea may rapidly lead to it, as can vomiting. If vomiting, diarrhea, and fever all occur concurrently, dehydration will develop quickly, as will electrolyte loss, that is the loss of critical blood buffering components such as potassium, sodium, chloride, and bicarbonate. This combination of fluid and electrolyte loss can be deadly.

Diabetics and/or individuals taking diuretics are at the highest risk of developing life-threatening dehydration. Laxative abuse, that is the chronic use of laxatives, may also precipitate it. Major symptoms of dehydration include:
• dry mouth or eyes
• lack of tearing
• dry skin
• constipation
• confusion
• agitation and/or hallucinations
• lack of urination or little urination

Dehydration mainly occurs in the elderly and in small children. If these individuals become sick, it is a good rule to evaluate them often for signs of dehydration.

Dehydration combat kit
• water (mineral water is best)
• juices (non-citrus juices such as grape, peach, pear, apricot, papaya, and fresh vegetable are well tolerated and highly nourishing)
• clear soup or soup broths provide both fluid and electrolytes
• high water foods are exceptional for replenishing; eat watermelon, cantaloupe, honeydew melon, radishes, turnips, red sweet peppers, tomatoes, and cucumbers.
• sea salt — once the fluids are replenished this helps prevent water loss. Note: some dehydration is due to salt deficiency, and water balance cannot be maintained unless salt is administered.
• premium grade royal jelly — strengthens the adrenal glands, which are responsible for fluid balance.
• oil of rosemary and sage (also for strengthening the adrenal glands) — take 5 drops of each twice daily.

Things to avoid
• all sources of caffeine (it is a dehydrating agent)

- alcoholic beverages (they are diuretics)
- antihistamines and anti-pain drugs, including aspirin, ibuprofen, and acetaminophen

Dengue fever

This disease is caused by a virus. It is transmitted by a mosquito that lives almost exclusively in the tropics. However, the mosquito is an inhabitant of the Southern United States and has been found in significant numbers in Louisiana and Texas. In fact, an outbreak of this disease, affecting some 750,000 individuals, occurred in Texas in the 1920s.

As described in *JAMA* dengue fever is currently an epidemic in Central America. However, it could strike in epidemic proportions in North America, particularly in the Deep South. It should always be suspected as a possible cause of illness for those becoming sick after traveling in the tropics, particularly Central and South America. In fact, any traveler to Central/South America, as well as Southeast Asia, could contract it.

Dengue fever is one of several hemorrhagic fevers which occur frequently in the tropics. It is sort of a milder form of Ebola. One helpful fact in establishing the diagnosis is that the mosquito which transmits it usually bites during the day. Usually, dengue is represented by a disconcerting illness that dissipates within two weeks. However, the hemorrhagic type is a killer, and up to one in five die.

Modern medicine claims that nothing can be done to prevent these deaths and that "supportive" care is the only option. Do not make this assumption. The condition should be treated aggressively with vitamins and herbs that block the damage, plenty of fluids, as well as with natural anti-infective agents.

An outbreak of dengue in the United States is a realistic issue for Southerners. This is particularly true since Hurricane Mitch. As described by the *Chicago Tribune* (January, 1999) hundreds of Honduran/Nicaraguan refugees are crossing the border daily, and all potentially harbor the disease. It is certain that such refugees harbor a wide range of diseases contracted in the aftermath of the hurricane. An outbreak within this population could rapidly spread to the indigenous peoples. With dengue this would likely develop in the summer, since the disease is spread by mosquito bites, and this is when these pests are most active.

Dengue combat kit
• oil of oregano SuperStrength — take large amounts; 3 or 4 drops under the tongue every few minutes; 20 drops (which fills a gelatin capsule nicely) internally every hour if necessary. Rub the oil on the face and buttocks (a means of rapid absorption into the blood through the skin). Or, take Oreganol gelcaps, about 2 twice daily.
• oil of cumin — 20 drops (i.e. fill a gelatin or vegi-cap) three or more times daily.
• oil of lavender — topically rub liberally all over the body. Inhale into the nostrils and rub on the inside of the nose with a Q-tip. Take 2 drops under the tongue occasionally.
• Flavin-C — take 2 to 4 capsules every hour in an attempt to halt hemorrhaging.
• oil of rosemary — 10 drops twice daily.
• juice of raw onion (yellow onion is preferable) — drink a cup or more per day. It may be enhanced with radish juice.
• Oregamax capsules — as many as can be swallowed.

Foods that help
• vitamin C rich juices may help curb hemorrhaging; otherwise, rest the system of food
• raw honey — useful for curbing diarrhea

Things to avoid
• blood thinners, including aspirin
• non-steroidal antiinflammatory drugs (i.e. arthritis/pain medication)
• stagnant water: if possible, be sure to eliminate all sources of it near the home, since this is where mosquitoes breed.

Dermatitis
This is defined as inflammation and/or irritation of the skin. Dermatitis is a rash, which often occurs on the skin in circumscribed patches. In extreme cases the entire body may be enveloped in it.

There are dozens of types of dermatitis, and there are just as many causes. The most common cause is allergic reaction. Reactions may be to foods, but the most likely culprits are chemicals. Dermatitis is an exceptionally frequent side effect of drugs. Foods which commonly provoke allergic dermatitis include milk products, refined sugar, chocolate, wheat, rye, and corn.

Dermatitis combat kit
• oil of oregano — dilute in extra virgin olive oil or cocoa butter and apply. If the region is too sensitive, take the oil internally, 10 or more drops daily. Internal consumption is the main method for eradicating chronic dermatitis.
• Oil of Bay Berry (top agent for wound healing and for aiding irritated skin) — rub gently on irritated skin twice or more daily.
• premium grade royal jelly (to acidify the skin and regenerate the adrenal glands) — take 4 or more capsules daily.
• Oregamax capsules — take 3 capsules twice daily.
• primrose or borage oil — take 6 or more capsules daily.

Things to avoid
• lye based soaps and detergents of any kind. Wash clothes in hot water; add 10 or more drops of oil of oregano and/or oil of lavender; use baking soda or other non-caustic washing agents.
• milk products, apple juice, and citrus fruit
• refined sugar, chocolate, and caffeinated beverages

Diabetes and diabetic attacks
Rarely found in primitive societies, diabetes is the scourge of the Western world. It afflicts tens of millions of Americans. It is one of the top five causes of death nationally.

This is a disease of poor diet. With diabetes, the human body is unable to properly metabolize food, especially sugar. However, infection may be a contributing factor. Yeast and fungal infections rampage within diabetics.

If diabetics suffer blood sugar attacks, they must be fed. However, candy bars are not the answer. They should be given food; certainly, fruit or fruit juice will suffice to prevent fatality. Yet, blood sugar balancing herbs, such as extracts of cumin, cilantro, coriander, and artichoke, work equally as well as the sugar. Grape, carob, or pomegranate molasses are superb alternatives to sugar as emergency aids. However, again, it is best to improve the body's ability to control the blood sugar levels in order to avoid catastrophes. For instance, red sour grape (Resvitanol) provides natural chromium, direly needed for blood sugar regulation. Nutri-Sense contains natural thiamine and niacin, which are crucial for proper sugar metabolism.

Diabetes combat kit
• oil of cumin — this is of utmost importance; take 10 to 20 drops three times daily in juice or water.
• crushed fenugreek/cumin/coriander capsules (HerbSorb caps) — take 2 or more capsules with each meal.
• oil of myrtle — take 5 drops twice daily.
• oil of cilantro/coriander — take 5 to 10 drops with each meal.
• oil of oregano — 2 or more drops daily under the tongue. Also, 2 to 5 drops daily in juice or water.
• Oregamax capsules — take 2 or 3 twice daily.
• Nutri-Sense protein/B drink mix (made from nutrient-rich rice bran, polish, flax, etc.) — take 3 heaping tablespoons in juice, milk, or water as an anti-diabetic B vitamin nourishing agent.

Foods that help
• artichokes
• cumin seed
• cilantro leaves
• sea salt (add to food liberally; salt doesn't cause diabetes, but sugar does)

Things to avoid
• chocolate as well as all foods containing refined sugar
• refined flour, rice, barley, oats, and corn meal
• orange, pear, apricot, and apple juice
• pancakes, waffles, bread, and pastries

Diaper rash

This is not simply a rash; it is an infection of the skin, usually caused by yeasts. The baby may be a carrier for yeasts and may have vaginal and/or intestinal overgrowth. It is best to avoid drugs in children and utilize natural agents such as Lactobacillus and antifungal spices. Acidophilus bacteria and other normal flora inhibit the growth of yeasts.

Edible herbs with antiseptic power are the other alternative. Research by Cornell University, published in 1998, documents how certain edible herbs, particularly onion, garlic, and wild oregano, exert valuable antifungal actions. These herbs are safe for pregnant and/or nursing mothers. Plus, in the proper form they are safe for infants. Oregamax is a wild oregano, garlic, onion formula available for all ages. It also contains an edible unique wild mountainous berry called *Rhus coriaria* (mountain sumac, unrelated to poison sumac). Wild oregano is the main active ingredient. A study published in the *International Journal of Food Microbiology* found that wild oregano in an amount less than 1% completely killed all fungi tested against it. In the Mediterranean the Oregamax formula is consumed by children of all ages. For children old enough to eat solids merely mix the contents of two or more capsules per day in food to ward off yeast/fungus infections. For younger infants mix the Oregamax into raw honey or cereal; one or two capsules daily should suffice. Breast feeding mothers may take the Oregamax, 6 or more capsules daily, to benefit the infant. The point is wild oregano, as well as garlic, onion, and mountain sumac, are foods. What's more, these herbs are safer for human use than many of the substances freely given to children such as aspirin, acetaminophen, and even soda pop. However, do not give raw garlic to infants; it is too caustic. What's more, commercial oregano is irradiated and contains residues of thermonuclear ions. Thus, it would not be appropriate to give to infants (or anyone else). The oregano in Oregamax is entirely wild and is never irradiated. It may be taken for any of the wide range of fungal infections afflicting infants and children. Oregamax may be purchased at health food stores and/or pharmacies, or to order direct call 1-800-243-5242.

If the mother is breast feeding, she too may require treatment with antifungal agents and/or acidophilus cultures. Breast-feeding mothers should avoid consuming drugs whenever possible, since these chemicals will be transferred into the breast milk and passed on to the baby. Yet, the same is true of natural substances, even natural bacteria. Once the friendly bacteria are ingested, they populate the mucous membranes of the gut. Additionally, they may be absorbed into the bloodstream. From here they are concentrated in breast milk. Noxious microbes may also be transported from the bowel into the blood and end up in the milk. These facts emphasize the importance of treating both the mother and the infant in preventing Candida overgrowth.

Breast milk is a derivative of the mother's diet, and whatever she eats/drinks and whatever medicine she takes will be in it. Thus, breast feeding mothers, as well as infants, should strictly avoid the intake of drugs if possible.

Care should be taken on how to cleanse the involved skin of diaper rash. A thorough rinsing with lukewarm water usually suffices; add a small amount of a gentle type of essential oil to a warm wash cloth (Oil of Bay Berry, oil of rosemary, oil of myrtle, etc.). Avoid using harsh soaps, as they usually cause further irritation. The skin is acidic and most soaps are basic, and they tend to alter it towards a basic pH. This encourages the growth of fungi as well as pathogenic bacteria.

Diaper rash combat kit

• oil of oregano (an excellent antifungal) — dilute this by adding 5 drops in a tablespoon of olive oil; apply as needed. However, before using it on sensitive baby skin be sure to read the label carefully. DO NOT use aromatherapy oregano oil or *THYMUS CAPITUS*, that is the so called full strength or undiluted types. These may burn the baby's sensitive skin. It may not be a permanent burn, but, nonetheless, such a reaction should be avoided. It is possible that some of these inferior types of oregano oils might contain synthetic ingredients. Be certain the product used contains only natural oil of oregano extracted from the wild plant. Use only the type(s) emulsified in extra virgin olive oil (must say on the label *guaranteed wild* oregano oil, wild crafted, or 100%

wild, i.e. North American Herb & Spice, Source Naturals, Physician's Strength, Oreganum, etc.).
- Oregamax capsules (for the mother or child) — take one or more capsules daily.
- Oil of Bay Berry — apply to the irritated skin as needed.
- oil of lavender — apply to the irritated skin as needed.

Things to avoid
- refined sugar and candies of all types
- harsh soaps
- perfumed diapers

Diarrhea

Of all sudden illnesses, this is one of the worst to develop. This is because uncontrolled diarrhea may rapidly lead to severe weakness, dehydration, perhaps death. In fact, diarrhea causes untold millions of deaths world wide, especially in primitive countries.

Uncontrolled diarrhea is particularly disastrous in children. In fact, diarrhea is perhaps the primary cause of childhood illness, and it kills millions of children every year, primarily in poor countries. While in a catastrophic circumstance diarrheal illnesses pose potentially serious problems, nationally, fewer than 1,000 children die every year as a result of this condition. The fact is virtually all childhood deaths from diarrhea are preventable.

If diarrhea afflicts large numbers of people, there must be an obvious source for the infection. Either the food or water must be contaminated. Attempt to determine what this source is to avoid re-infection. Germs which commonly cause food/water borne epidemics include hepatitis viruses, E. coli, Salmonella, Shigella, Camphylobacter, trichinella (pork worms), Vibrio (the cause of cholera), Giardia, and Cryptosporidium. All can cause fulminant life-threatening diarrhea.

Diarrhea combat kit
- raw honey — consume as much as necessary, up to a pound per day (diabetics must omit this one).
- oil of oregano — a few drops under the tongue repetitively. Also, take a few drops or Oreganol caps internally daily.

- oil of myrtle (anti-cramp) — take 5 drops two or three times daily.
- Juice of Oregano — drink 2 ounces three times daily or more often if necessary.
- HerbSorb (Eastern aromatic spice and intestinal tonic formula) — take 3 capsules several times daily.

Foods that help
- raw honey is easy on the gut
- clear meat or chicken broths
- onion/garlic broth
- ginger root tea

Things to avoid
- chocolate and refined sugar
- solid foods
- apple and orange juice

Diphtheria

According to Miriam Tucker, senior writer for *Family Practice News*, diphtheria is "alive and well"...in the United States. Thus, unfortunately, this scary disease has yet to be erased despite immunizations. In fact, modern medicine bragged that the organism was essentially eliminated from the populous. Yet, as described by Dr. W. A. Orenstein in *Family Practice News*, June 15, 1998, an epidemic of this dreaded disease remains a significant possibility. Diphtheria is primarily a throat disorder, that is an infection of the throat by a bacteria. This bacteria not only invades the throat but also produces a potent toxin, diphtheria toxin, which can cause damage throughout the body. Because it is so rare in the United States, it may be easily missed. This increases the risks for a serious outbreak.

The typical symptom is a sore throat with a membranous tissue attached on the mucous membranes that develops beyond the tonsils. This membrane may extend all the way into the lungs. Other symptoms include swollen neck lymph nodes, low grade fever, chills, and hoarseness. Suspicion should be high for diphtheria if the typical symptoms develop in individuals traveling to Russia or the

Orient. While a diphtheria epidemic is unlikely, it is necessary to prepare for it, because, when it strikes, it is often deadly.

Diphtheria is an extremely dangerous illness. It requires immediate medical care. Physicians usually prescribe Erythromycin and/or penicillin for a 14 day period. Perhaps even more important in reversing the disease is the Diphtheria Antitoxin, which is effective especially if given early in the course. The latter is given as an injection. However, this is an experimental drug and is not routinely available in emergency rooms. It must be purchased by physicians or hospitals from the CDC by calling 1-404-639-2889.

Antibiotics alone may be insufficient to halt this disastrous infection, especially if an epidemic strikes. Antiseptic herbs, such as garlic, onion, and wild oregano, must also be relied upon. Oil of oregano can sterilize sewage, and diphtheria germs are a minor issue compared to that.

Diphtheria combat kit
* oil of oregano (SuperStrength is best) — take aggressively, 2 or more drops under the tongue every half hour or as often as necessary. Also, take 5 to 10 drops three times daily in juice or water.
* bromelain (antiinflammatory agent) — take 3 or more capsules three times daily on an empty stomach.
* Flavin-C — take 3 capsules four times daily.
* Oregamax capsules — take 3 capsules three times daily.
* Black seed-plus (aromatic antiseptic) — take 3 capsules twice daily.
* oil of wild lavender — rub on soles of feet, forehead, and chest

Foods that help
* papaya plus the seeds
* meat based broths with garlic and onion

Things to avoid
* all types of pop and milk products
* refined sugar in any form (it is immunosuppressive)

Diverticulitis (see also Constipation)

This is an inflammatory disorder of the colon, largely due to damage to the colon wall from straining at the stool. It can cause considerable pain and discomfort. Occasionally, it develops into a medical emergency, because the colon wall becomes infected with bacteria or parasites. This may lead to abscess formation. If this condition is untreated, the colon wall may rupture, causing life-threatening infections.

Diverticulitis combat kit
- wild oregano herb (Oregamax) — take 3 capsules twice daily.
- oil of oregano — take 2 drops under the tongue twice daily. Take also 5 drops in juice or water or 1 Oreganol cap 2x daily.
- oil of rosemary (for relaxing the intestinal walls) — take 5 drops in juice or water twice daily.
- Nutri-Sense protein/B vitamin drink mix — take 3 tablespoons in juice or water. Add a tablespoon of carob molasses and mix in a blender with frozen fruit. Very nourishing for the bowel, yet gentle.
- BromaZyme — take 2 capsules with each meal.

Things to avoid
- peanuts and other legumes
- nuts and seeds
- refined sugar, colas, pastries, and cookies
- white flour and foods made with flour

Dog bites

As incredible as it may seem over a million Americans are bitten by dogs every year. Some estimates place the number as high as 4.5 million, because many of the bites are never reported. The point is virtually anyone is likely to be bitten by a dog. The Postal Service is well aware of the scope of this dilemma, as thousands of mail carriers are included among the victims. However, children are the most common victims. Weiss and colleagues noted in *JAMA* that nearly one half of all children, that is tens of millions of individuals, suffer at least one dog bite during their life times. Unfortunately, a high percentage of these bites are on the face, neck, and head. Thus, dog bites are an enormous health issue in the United States, costing the country tens of millions of dollars. The extent of this problem is so vast that bites by other animals, including cats, must be considered relatively rare in comparison. In fact, human bites are possibly the second most common "animal" bite.

Any animal bite can become infected. Bites are a type of puncture wound, where contaminated secretions are injected deep into the tissues. The deeper a puncture is into the muscle, the greater is the risk for infection. Deep wounds receive less oxygen than superficial ones. Blood flow is greatest in the skin and least in the deep muscles. This reduced blood flow largely contributes to the high risk for infection in puncture wounds.

Dog bites notoriously become infected. Any dog bite which breaks the skin, no matter how superficial, can become infected. When their teeth puncture the skin, dog saliva is driven deep into the tissues. This saliva is loaded with germs. Dog lovers might find this difficult to believe, but it is true.

In the emergency rooms physicians advise patients to leave dog bites open and rarely suture them. Experience has proven that closing (suturing) the wound traps the infections within the tissues. Not only will the wound heal poorly if it is closed, but also potentially severe or even life-threatening infections may result.

Dog bite combat kit
• flush the wound liberally with clean water, hopefully clean saline water.
• oil of oregano — drizzle copious amounts throughout the wound.
• oil of lavender — add to wound and rub around the wound site; speeds healing.
• Royal Kick premium grade royal jelly — take to combat stress and strengthen the adrenal glands, 2 to 4 capsules every morning.
• bromelain — to reduce trauma and swelling, take 2 or more capsules twice daily on an empty stomach.
• Oil of Bay Berry — anti-pain; also speeds healing.

Drug overdose
Drugs are defined as cellular poisons. This makes them extremely dangerous to use unsupervised during crises. Drugs should only be dispensed under a doctor's direction. Even under a doctor's

direction they are dangerous. The *JAMA* reported in April, 1998, that over 100,000 individuals are killed and another 2.2 million harmed yearly by reactions from drugs, which are *properly* dispensed. This doesn't include the damage inflicted by improperly dispensed medications, which account for additional thousands of deaths and injuries. In fact, the research was skewed, because they reviewed only deaths due to properly prescribed medications. The number would likely triple if other drug induced disasters were included. What's more, millions of other individuals, perhaps as many as 5 million, suffer adverse reactions to non-prescription drugs every year. Computer crashes will accentuate this dilemma, since in today's hospitals and pharmacies drug dispensing is heavily computerized.

The consumption of prescription drugs by the public in an attempt to self-medicate is a dangerous practice. It is particularly ill-advised during disaster circumstances, when access to emergency medical care may be compromised. The point is it is likely to cause more harm than good. For instance, you develop a cough or sore throat, and you have left-over antibiotics from a previous prescription. You take those antibiotics on your own. Yet, if the problem is due to a herpes viral infection, mono, or a respiratory virus, you will likely aggravate and prolong the illness. What's more, you may create drug resistant germs that could cause long term illness and perhaps spread dangerously to the internal organs.

Children are highly vulnerable to the toxic effects of drugs. Non-prescription drugs and over-the-counter tablets are the primary causes of childhood poisoning. Incredibly, first on the list are multiple vitamins, which cause iron poisoning. However, perhaps even more insidious are antibiotics, which are the primary cause of prescription drug toxicity in children/infants. According to S. Knowles, reviewing data from Health Canada, fully 75% of all drug reactions in children under 16 were caused by antibiotics: over 20% were serious, that is they were capable of causing permanent damage and/or death. The reactions include severe rash, hives, diarrhea, swelling, and shock.

The liver is the organ responsible for detoxifying and removing harmful chemicals and thus bears the brunt of drug toxicity. Specifically, drugs damage the liver by depleting it of critical components, particularly vitamins and certain enzymes. The enzymes which are severely depleted are primarily glutathione and, to a lesser degree, superoxide dismutase. Glutathione depletion alone accounts for much of the drug induced damage. Therefore, agents which replenish glutathione do much to repair liver damage or prevent it from occurring. Top glutathione replenishing agents include N-acetyl cysteine (NAC), glutathione tablets, organic selenium, rosemary oil, cumin oil, oregano oil, and cilantro oil. Use only the edible oils emulsified in olive oil. Do not use aromatherapy grade essential oils, since they have not been screened for edibility. Do not use sodium selenite or selenious acid. These synthetic types of selenium may accentuate the chemical poisoning.

Another advantage of edible plant essential oils is that they may aid in restoring bile synthesis as well as stimulating the flow of bile. Drugs are stored in the bile producing portion of the liver and the ideal means to eliminate them is through the bile. Top bile stimulants include oils of fennel, lavender, cumin, rosemary, and oregano, with cumin being perhaps the most effective of these.

Certain herbs, such as milk thistle, beet extract, artichoke, and chlorella, are well respected liver detoxifying agents. However, they are far less potent than the edible essential oils in purging the liver of poisonous compounds.

Drug detoxification kit
- oil of cumin — take 10 to 20 drops three times daily.
- oil of rosemary — take 10 drops twice daily.
- oil of oregano — take 10 drops twice daily.
- oil of cilantro/coriander — take 10 or more drops twice daily.
- organically bound selenium — take 200 mcg every few hours until the toxicity is resolved (no more than one week on this dose). As a maintenance, take 400 mg daily.
- NAC — take 1000 mg per day.
- activated charcoal — actually absorbs the drug so it can be removed through the bowels.
- crude ascorbic acid/bioflavonoids (Flavin-C) — take 2 capsules every few hours until the toxicity is abated. Also, use regular vitamin C, about 1000 mg twice daily.

Foods that help
- artichokes, black radish, garlic, and onion
- beets and beet tops
- pure extra virgin olive oil plus vinegar (as a liver flush)

Note: anyone taking prescription drugs must see his/her physician before taking new items or altering the prescription.

Dry or irritated eyes

Dryness of the eyes is a classic symptom of nutritional deficiency. Vitamin A, zinc, and essential fatty acids are the missing nutrients, although vitamin B_2 deficiency may play a role. Essential fatty acids are a must for correcting this condition. Excellent sources include primrose and borage oils plus to a lesser degree flax oil. Vitamin A eye drops would be curative in the event of its deficiency, which is manifested by dry and/or inflamed eyes. Also, consume foods rich in vitamin A such as organic liver, fatty fish, and whole milk products. Be sure to take essential fatty acid supplements as well as cod liver oil, because in many cases the condition is too severe to rely on food sources alone. About nine capsules of primrose oil and a teaspoon of cod liver oil daily should suffice.

E. coli

This bacteria is a normal inhabitant of the bowel. It only causes problems if it overgrows or if it enters other regions such as the bladder, kidneys, and/or prostate. It was only rarely a problem prior to modern time. However, now it is a killer. This is because a number of mutant strains have been created by antibiotics. These mutant strains are highly aggressive and are capable of rapidly destroying human tissue. They essentially liquefy certain organs unless they can be quickly eliminated from the body.

No one can afford to have mutant E. coli in the body for long. It must be destroyed promptly. Unfortunately, no synthetic antibiotic is 100% capable of that. I have made it evident that natural substances, specifically oil of oregano, are capable of filling the void by killing noxious germs outright. A recent study performed by the University of Tennessee in concert with the FDA attempted to dispute these findings. However, unexpectedly, it was determined that a variety of natural compounds, particularly oil of oregano, killed the type of E. coli that contaminates food. Thus, natural antiseptics may well be lifesaving for this condition.

> *Case history:* a 17 year-old girl contracted severe diarrhea from mutant E. coli. The diarrhea was unstoppable; in fact, according to her mother the hospital sent her home to die. Her mother gave her one dose of oil of oregano, and the diarrhea stopped completely. This beautiful young lady is now totally healthy, but, just in case, she takes a drop or two of oil of oregano every day.

E. coli combat kit
• oil of oregano SuperStrength — bombard it; take 2 to 4 drops under the tongue frequently; take also 10 to 20 drops internally, as often as every hour. Reduce this amount to a maintenance level of 2 drops twice daily once the infestation is destroyed.
• wild oregano capsules (Oregamax) — take 3 capsules three times daily.
• oil of cumin — take 10 drops twice daily.
• oil of cilantro/coriander — take 10 drops twice daily.
• Lactobacillus supplement (take also as a daily preventive)
• raw garlic — chew on cloves to tolerance.

Foods that help
• raw garlic and onion (add to foods frequently)
• onion juice — one or more cups daily
• papaya and kiwi fruit
• ginger root in food or in hot water (as a tea)

Earache and/or infection
Ear infections are one of the most difficult dilemmas faced by parents today. The incidence of this condition has risen in children dramatically over the last fifty years. Adults rarely develop them.

Nearly 50% of the incidents where parents think their child has an ear infection, he/she doesn't. This is according to the latest research by Dr. Weiss and colleagues from Phoenix's Children's

Hospital. Perhaps even more astounding is the fact that these orthodox M.D.s categorically state that a large percentage of earaches completely resolve without treatment. What's more, when a true ear infection does occur, as many as 40% of them may be due to organisms other than bacteria such as viruses and fungi, both of which are immune to antibiotics.

When parents are confronted with earaches or infections in their children they often become concerned that the infection will spread from the inner ear to the brain, which is in close proximity. Yet, what parents fail to realize is that a huge percentage of ear aches are caused by toxic reactions to foods, not germs. However, bacteria often invade the ear canal secondarily as a result of the allergic reaction. In a crisis it may be cumbersome to avoid potentially allergenic foods. Combine this with stress, exposure to the elements, and communicable diseases, and earaches can become a significant dilemma.

The inner and middle ear cavities are in close proximity to the brain. So are the sinuses, roots of the teeth, and eye sockets. Infections in any of these regions could theoretically spread to the brain. Infection of the brain in children is relatively rare, but when it occurs, it is frequently fatal. These infections include meningitis, encephalitis, and brain abscess. However, an incredibly small percentage of cases of ear infections lead to brain or spinal cord infection. The vast majority of cases of meningitis, encephalitis, and brain abscesses are caused as a consequence of other factors, including poor hygiene, blood poisoning, animal bites, insect bites, pneumonia, and surgery (and its complications). People should be equally if not more concerned about these factors as they are about ear infections.

The current approach is to aggressively treat ear infections with prescription medicines. Frequently, doctors prescribe repeated doses of potent drugs, like broad spectrum antibiotics, cortisone, and codeine. Antibiotics are over-prescribed by pediatricians for virtually all childhood illnesses. This is because doctors are afraid of being sued. Children, particularly infants, are easily overdosed by such medicines, and numerous side effects may result. Antibiotics are far from innocuous. In fact, they may occasionally cause life-threatening reactions.

Antibiotic therapy creates its own group of illnesses. These illnesses include chronic candidiasis, vaginitis, cystitis, chronic serous otitis media, irritable bowel syndrome, pseudomembranous colitis, and food intolerance.

Children are also over medicated with anti-fever agents like aspirin and Tylenol. Other drugs are given for pain such as opium derivatives, i.e. codeine. Drugs containing codeine, should never be given to children without medical supervision. The ill effects of this drug upon respiration are of particular concern. If lung function is depressed, less oxygen will be available for the tissues, and the results may be catastrophic. Impaired function of the immune system will result, and the function of the brain, the body's number one oxygen consumer, may be seriously impaired. If this respiratory depression occurs for a prolonged period, seizures and/or coma may result. Additionally, the systemic physiological depression induced by codeine increases the tendency for infections to spread. As a result, a self-limiting disease can be turned into a fatal one.

Antibiotics are highly destructive to bowel bacteria, particularly the friendly bacteria. They are less able to develop resistance to antibiotics than pathogens, and, thus, they are routinely destroyed in vast numbers as a result of even modest dosages. The destruction of the friendly bacteria encourages the growth of pathogenic organisms. Yeasts grow prolifically as a consequence of destruction of the normal flora, since the latter secrete a variety of substances which inhibit the growth of fungi. Thus, antibiotics both cause and aggravate yeast infections.

Antibiotics negatively affect immunity. They impair white blood cell function. Evidence exists that they cause a significant reduction in the *phagocytic index*, a measurement of the ability of white blood cells to destroy microbes. The reduction in the immune potential encourages the development of opportunistic infections, the very thing that doctors are attempting to cure.

Prolonged use of potent medicines increases patients' risks for developing a variety of ailments. Infants and children are significantly more vulnerable to these ill effects than are adults. Do not over-medicate your children.

Ear infection combat kit

• oil of oregano — this may be all you need; rub on the outer ear or the skin behind the ear. Also, take a drop or as necessary daily under the tongue, two or more times daily.
• oil of lavender — rub on face, chest, soles of feet, and outer ear
• Oil of Bay Berry — rub on face, chest, outer ear, buttocks, and soles of feet. For tender skin dilute with olive oil.
• Oregamax capsules — take as many capsules as possible, up to 4 per day. If the child is too small to swallow, open and add to bottle or food.

Things to avoid

• milk products
• white sugar, chocolate, and candy
• apple and orange juice

Ebola

Ebola has developed in the United States. This is what inspired the book *Hot Zone* and its resulting movie, *Outbreak*. Indeed, like the book and movie the USA outbreak was monkey induced. However, none of the individuals who were infected died. This is because the monkey virus was a weakened mutant of the more severe human type.

The human type rapidly devastates anyone in its path. As described in *Hippocrates Magazine* during the largest outbreak of Ebola yet in Africa nine out of ten individuals died. The death is gruesome but not always quick. There may be up to two weeks of intense suffering before the ultimate demise. Death is usually via organ liquefaction. If Ebola strikes, don't give up hope. Use the Ebola combat kit as aggressively as possible to save your life and the lives of others.

Ebola combat kit

• oil of oregano (SuperStrength is best) — take massive amounts, like 5 drops under the tongue every 15 minutes and 20 drops internally every hour. Rub on soles of feet and chest.
• oil of bay leaf — take 10 or more drops twice daily in juice or water.
• oil of cumin — take 20 drops several times daily in juice or water.
• Flavin-C — take as much as possible to impede blood vessel destruction; consume an entire bottle a day, if necessary.

• red grape powder (Resvitanol) — the bulk form is ideal; take up to a heaping teaspoon every hour.
• oil of lavender and/or Oil of Bay Berry — rub all over the body if necessary (skin application may be lifesaving, especially if the gut is compromised).
• oil of myrtle — rub vaginally and/or insert a gelatin capsule filled with the oil into the rectum; the flavonoids are anti-bleeding.
• BromaZyme — take 2 capsules several times daily.

Foods that help
• onion juice (yellow onions are best) — drink as much as can be consumed
• raw garlic — eat as many cloves as can be stomached
• raw honey — eat it by the cupful
• carob molasses — well digested and an ideal source of nourishment for fighting the infection, 1 or 2 teaspoons daily

Eczema

This condition is a type of chronic inflammation of the skin. For years no one was sure what caused it. Many presumed it was due to allergies or sensitivity to chemicals in soap, etc.

The medical profession has erred greatly in its approach to this illness. All manner of creams and ointments have been dispensed, largely to no avail. This failure is due to the fact that eczema is primarily an internal disorder, i.e. the cause is systemic. It was Rosenberg and colleagues at the University of Tennessee who first made the determination: germs are the cause of eczema. They found that the eczema lesions and psoriatic blotches contained a fungus as well as staph and/or strep. Apparently, the germs arise from inside the body, that is from within the bowel, and infect the skin secondarily. Thus, the only way to resolve this disorder is to eradicate the infection *internally*. In other words, killing the fungus and/or bacteria is the objective. The same is true of psoriasis.

Certain substances, notably pure essential oils in a carrier base, may be helpful rubbed externally. Ideally, use a combined approach of internal plus external therapies.

Eczema combat kit
- oil of oregano — take 2 drops under the tongue twice daily. Also, take 5 or more drops twice daily internally. For tough cases the SuperStrength may be necessary.
- oil of myrtle or Bay Berry — rub externally on irritated skin or eczema lesions to tolerance.
- Oregamax capsules — take 3 or more capsules twice daily.
- Juice of Oregano — take an ounce or more daily with meals.

Things to avoid
- caffeine, soda pop, and chocolate
- refined sugar and corn syrup

Emotionally distressed child
This covers a wide range of conditions wherein a toddler or child is distressed, that is out of control. No one can afford to deal with this nerve wracking situation, whether in everyday life or a disaster. The answers are found in nutrients, herbs, spices, and aromatic plant oils.

Emotional distress combat kit
- oil of lavender (wild type) — rub topically on the chest, especially at night. Also, rub on soles of feet and buttocks.
- oil of sage in olive oil — highly calming, rub on face, chest, and especially soles of feet and mid-lower back (adrenal reflex).
- Royal Kick (premium quality royal jelly) — 2 or more capsules in the morning.
- B complex — take one tablet twice daily.
- Nutri-Sense — a superior, natural source of B vitamins and fatty acids, take 2 tablespoons twice daily in juice, milk, or water.
- Essence of Orange Blossom or White Coffee— add a tablespoon or more to juice or hot tea; drink once or twice daily.
- oil of oregano (rub on chest and soles of feet)
- primrose oil — take as directed or 6 capsules daily.

Foods that help
- salted roasted nuts (MSG-free)
- peanut butter with salt (high in B vitamins and protein)
- sliced turkey meat (high in tryptophan)

- fatty fish, especially salmon

Things to avoid
- candy, sugar, cookies, or sweets of any kind
- pop and other caffeinated/sugary drinks
- synthetic food dyes or flavorings

Emphysema

If there is a disease of torment, it is emphysema. In this condition the individual is literally suffocating to death in his/her own secretions. Life with emphysema is miserable and death by it even worse.

Emphysema is largely due to toxic chemical damage to the lungs. Thus, it is particularly common in industrial workers and cigarette smokers. Yet, it is also prolific in non-smokers who live in highly polluted regions like Los Angeles, New York City, and Chicago. While the medical profession regards emphysema as incurable, the lungs have an immense capacity to regenerate. Nutrients needed for lung cell regeneration include beta carotene, vitamins C and E, flavonoids, zinc, and selenium. Essential oils also assist cellular repair.

Emphysema may also be caused by chronic infection. Molds and bacteria readily infect the lungs, causing tissue damage. If the infection is eradicated, the breathing improves significantly. Destruction of infection is key to remission of this disorder.

Nutritional deficiency is another major factor. The key deficient nutrients are vitamins A, C, and E as well as pantothenic acid, essential fatty acids, and phospholipids.

Emphysema combat kit
- oil of oregano (SuperStrength may be required) — take 2 drops under the tongue two or more times daily.
- oil of rosemary — take 2 to 5 drops twice daily in juice or water. Also, rub on chest and under nose.
- Oil of Bay Berry — rub all over the body, particularly on the face, chest, and soles of the feet.
- Flavin-C — take 2 or more capsules twice daily.
- vitamin E — take 1200 I.U. daily of a high quality natural source vitamin E (mixed tocopherols or tocotrienols).

• beta carotene — take 50,000 I.U. of a natural source mixed carotenoid supplement daily. Also, take vitamin A (as fish oil extract or cod liver oil), 20,000 I.U. daily.
• Oregamax capsules — take 3 capsules or more twice daily (an excellent lung tonic).**Note:** essential oils and wild herbs are more aggressive in aiding the lung function than vitamins. Crude sources of flavonoids, such as Flavin-C, are also highly useful.

Foods that help
• squash, pumpkin, sweet potatoes

Things to avoid
• any contact with smoke as well as moldy or damp rooms

Encephalitis
This is defined simply as inflammation of the brain and the linings around it. It is nearly always virally induced. It is life threatening.

Usually, this condition develops as a consequence of insect bites, mostly mosquitoes, however, ticks can also cause it. World wide, mosquitoes cause millions of cases of encephalitis, which these insects contract from the blood of rodents and other wild animals (as well as humans). Encephalitis may also develop in the aftermath of common viral illnesses; measles, chickenpox, mumps, and viral pneumonia may all result in it. It frequently develops after natural catastrophes, like floods. Recently (September, 1999), a bizarre virus began attacking individuals throughout American. Called the West Nile virus, it infected hundreds of individuals throughout the country. This virus will likely cause a national encephalitis epidemic, leading to hundreds of deaths. Without substantial protection thousands of individuals could die. Protect yourself with the power of anti-viral edible essential oils. For instance, one study showed that oil of wild oregano disintegrated viruses, a power not found in drugs.

Encephalitis combat kit
• oil of oregano — take 2 drops under the tongue often, like every hour; also, take 5 drops twice daily or (2 to 4 Oreganol).
• oil of lavender — rub on face, under nose, on scalp, buttocks, and soles of feet.
• oil bay leaf — take 5 drops twice daily.

- Flavin-C — take 3 capsules three times daily.
- Oregamax capsules — take 9 or more capsules daily.
- Oil of Bay Berry — rub anywhere on the body.
- Juice of Rosemary — take 2 or more ounces daily.
- Black seed-plus — take 3 capsules twice daily.

Foods that help
- squash (especially butternut), pumpkin, and sweet potatoes
- watercress, arugula, spinach, and parsley
- garlic/onion meat based broths

Endometriosis

This is an inflammatory condition of the female organs. It can afflict any of the pelvic female organs or glands, especially the ovaries, uterus, and fallopian tubes. It can even attack abdominal organs, like the bowel.

Endometriosis occurs when fluids from the uterus spill into aberrant areas, like the abdominal cavity, causing massive inflammation. The conduit for this is the fallopian tubes, the same ones that transport the eggs. Infection is the most likely cause for this condition. However, hormonal insufficiency is another major cause, that is poor output of natural steroids such as progesterone, estrogen, and cortisol.

Endometriosis combat kit
- oil of oregano — take 2 drops under the tongue twice daily.
- premium grade royal jelly (Royal Kick, very important) — take 4 to 6 capsules in the a.m.
- oil of myrtle — rub on the vaginal walls twice daily.
- oil of rosemary — take 5 to 10 drops twice daily.
- PureKelp — take 2 to 4 capsules daily in the morning.
- Nutri-Sense drink mix — take 3 T. daily in juice or water.
- Resvitanol — take 2 capsules twice daily.

Foods that help
- raw sunflower seeds
- fatty fish, especially salmon

Things to avoid
- refined sugar, candy, cookies, etc.
- chocolate, tea, iced tea, and coffee
- hydrogenated and partially hydrogenated oils
- sex during menses

Exhaustion

Exhaustion is something virtually everyone has experienced. It is usually caused by severe stress, physical exertion, or disease. Nutritional deficiency also results in fatigue/exhaustion. To survive in today's rather hostile world it is required to have a full bank of energy. Exhaustion negatively affects the individual in every aspect of life, in relationships, work, and enjoyment. There is no need to be exhausted. By taking strength producing remedies it is possible to have plenty of energy, perhaps an excess of it, quickly.

Exhaustion combat kit
- Royal Kick (premium grade royal jelly) — take 4 to 6 capsules every morning. If necessary, take another 2 to 4 at noon.
- Juice of Oregano (a strength tonic) — take an ounce twice daily.
- Hercules Strength — take 3 capsules twice daily.
- Oregamax capsules — take 2 or more twice daily.
- sage tea — make a tea by adding a tablespoon of Juice of Sage to a cup of hot water; drink once or twice daily.
- Nutri-Sense drink mix — take 3 tablespoons every morning in milk, juice, or water. Add to shakes, smoothies, cereals, or soups.

Foods that help
- salted roasted nuts
- roasted beef, turkey, or chicken (rich in carnitine, an energizing nutrient)

Exposure to the elements (see also Frostbite; Cold exposure)

Inevitably, this will develop as a consequence of a major disaster. Body temperature fluctuations, either too hot (heat intolerance) or too cold (hypothermia), are among the primary problems associated with exposure. Exposure can rapidly lead to physical damage, particularly in the elderly or very young.

Hypothermia, that is abnormally low body temperature, is the most life threatening consequence of exposure. Every year, tens of thousands of individuals, mostly the poor and homeless, suffer from it.

Exposure means the individual is exposed to potentially dangerous elements, that is to poor weather, excessive heat, and, particularly, to excessive cold and wet. Cold wet weather is particularly dangerous, especially if the individual has no shelter. Such exposure can rapidly lead to respiratory distress and/or infection, which may prove fatal.

Cold exposure combat kit
• oil of oregano — rub on face, hands, and feet to produce heat. Take 2 drops under the tongue twice or more daily.
• Royal Kick — to strengthen the adrenal glands, take 4 to 6 capsules every morning. For severe cold exposure take extra doses.
• Flavin-C — take 2 to 4 capsules twice daily.
• cayenne pepper — take 1/4 teaspoon or 1 or 2 capsules twice daily with juice or food.
• oil of sage and/or Juice of Sage — add to hot water and drink as a highly invigorating tea; a tremendous tonic for improving cold tolerance and reversing cold injury, including frostbite.
• wild strawberry leaf tea (WildPower Tea) — drink one or two cups daily.
• Black seed-plus — take 2 capsules twice daily to speed metabolism.
• PureKelp (for stimulating the thyroid gland) — take 4 to 6 capsules every morning.

Foods that help against cold
• salmon, albacore tuna, sardines, herring plus the juice
• meat broths rich in fat, onion, and garlic
• sea salt and salted foods
• hot spicy soups and sauces
• sea weed or miso soup

Heat exposure combat kit
• Royal Kick — good for too hot or too cold, this strengthens adrenal action; take 4 capsules twice daily or more often during extreme exposure.
• Flavin-C — crude vitamin C plus flavonoids greatly enhances heat tolerance; take 2 or more capsules several times daily.

Foods that help against heat
- watermelon and cantaloupe
- parsley and cilantro
- radishes and turnips
- salted dried meat, fish, or poultry
- meat based broths (garlic and onion added)

Note: interestingly, salt and salted (healthy) foods are helpful in building strength both in cold and heat exposure.

Fainting

Few people realize that smelling salts were originally based on using essential oils as the active ingredients. This is because certain essential oils are such profound sensory activating agents that they will wake up just about anyone.

Fainting may be caused by a number of diseases. However, usually the cause is innocuous such as sudden bouts of fear or anxiety or low blood sugar. Regardless of the cause "essential oil smelling salts" should be administered.

Fainting combat kit
- oil of bay leaf — rub on face and under nose as well as on the chest.
- oil of rosemary — rub on face and adrenal reflex in the mid lower back. Rub also on soles of feet. Give 2 or 3 drops under the tongue.
- oil of lavender — rub on face, under nose, on buttocks, and soles of the feet. Apply near or around nostrils.
- Oil of myrtle — rub on the face and spine or around the nostrils.

Fever

Parents, don't lose your minds over fevers. This is a natural process by which the body destroys germs. Everyone knows that heat kills germs. Fever by itself will only rarely harm or kill a human. In other words, it is not the fever that does so. It is the consequence of fever: dehydration and/or internal toxicity. As long as their is plenty of fluid in the body to buffer or insulate against high temperatures and to aid the body in the removal of toxins, fever is harmless.

In the event of high fever be sure to constantly push the fluids. Use cool compresses on the face and forehead. Avoid using anti-fever drugs. They are the primary cause of organ damage. Such drugs should only be consumed as a last resort, when all else fails. Instead, utilize substances which help naturally break fevers. The most effective of these are the essential oils.

Fever Combat Kit
• oil of oregano — usually, rapidly breaks fever. Take internally and rub topically.
• oil of lavender — a tremendous topical aid; helps cool skin and also breaks fever.
• oil of rosemary — a natural coolant; take internally or rub topically.
• wild oregano capsules (Oregamax) — take 2 or more capsules every four hours to strengthen immunity and dissipate heat.
• ginger — slice fresh ginger and add to hot water as a tea.
• Essence of Orange Blossom — cooling, yet effective in normalizing heat transfer. Add one or more tablespoons to hot water and drink as a tea.

It seems ironic that hot spices actually help dissipate heat. They accomplish this by stimulating metabolism and by forcing excess heat through the skin. This is readily apparent by anyone who eats hot spicy food. Often, the individual becomes hot and sweaty; this is the dissipation of heat through the skin. Thus, if you make chicken soup for fevers or infections, make it spicy.

Fire ants
These insects are not natural inhabitants of the United States, originating instead in South America. However, now they inhabit nearly all of the Southern states. Fire ants are feared, because their bites are intensely painful. What's more, bites occurring in highly allergic individuals and/or individuals who have been bitten previously may cause life-threatening shock. Typical symptoms of

the bites include pain, itching, swelling, redness, and, for allergic individuals, constricted breathing, shock, and collapse.

The editors of *USA Today* (1998) succinctly describe the fire ant epidemic, stating that these ants "kill, maim, and blind." Perhaps as much as one fifth of the land mass in the United States is contaminated by these pests, notably the entire states of South Carolina, Georgia, Florida, Alabama, Mississippi, Louisiana, and parts of Texas, North Carolina, and Tennessee. Recently, southern California (Orange County) has become infested. What's more, the ants are expanding northward several miles each year.

The fire ant is a tropical ant, the demonic man eating type of the movies. Unfortunately, it has efficiently adapted to our southern climate. What is perhaps more ominous is the fact that, perhaps through breeding with local ants, fire ants have adapted to cold weather, making their spread to unsuspecting Northern states virtually imminent.

Fire ants are vicious. In the wild they kill newborn deer and baby birds. They may attack adult farm animals. They have no fear of large creatures, after all, they are immigrants from the land of big game (i.e. South America/Africa). They are a serious menace to small children. Dozens of Americans have been killed by these ants, some of them, as described by Richard de Shazo, a director at the University of Mississippi Medical Center, Jackson, Mississippi, being literally "eaten alive."

The reason for their terror and toxicity isn't because of their bites per se: it is because of the highly poisonous venom they secrete when they bite. The venom itself usually doesn't kill humans. However, if an individual is allergic to it, shock and death may rapidly result.

Fire ants are learning to live indoors. For instance, in Florida they routinely enter homes in search for food. Different than normal ants, they will crawl on children (and adults) and bite them. Parents often have to scrape them off and then deal with a stinging itching lesion(s). If fire ants succeed at colonizing homes, they could be found in virtually every region of the United States, a disaster of unprecedented proportions.

The fire ant venom causes burning pain. This usually leads to intense itching, swelling, redness, hives, and pustule formation.

In an individual with multiple bites allergic shock may develop, leading to collapse, unconsciousness, and perhaps death. The biggest problem is with Northerners. They are unaware of the crisis, and, thus, when visiting the South take no precautions. Often, they don't even realize that the ants are the culprit; they may think it is "hives" or "food allergy." Or, they rush to the emergency room, deathly ill, while having no clue that they were stung by ants.

Fire ant combat kit
• oil of oregano — apply to bites; take 2 drops under the tongue every hour until resolved.
• Oil of Bay Berry or oil of bay — apply to bite region.
• raw garlic — crush and apply to bites.
• raw onion — crush and apply to bites.
• BromaZyme — take 2 to 3 capsules every hour until resolved.
Note: when attacked by a horde of ants it is difficult to react or think. However, if possible, attack them back with an oregano oil concoction. Grab a spray bottle and add a few ounces of hot water. Add a bottle or whatever amount is available of oil of oregano. Pump spray in a fine or medium mist directly at the ants. If no oil of oregano is available, crush a few cloves of garlic and add this to the water. These agents are so hot that they will damage the ants' sensors, and they will either fall off or die.

Fleas
No one could believe that a human could have fleas, yet, infestation by these insects afflicts thousands of Americans every year. Many individuals are unaware that fleas can't fly; they are hopping insects and infect individuals by jumping on them and burrowing into the skin.

Fleas can cause serious disease. They transport the Plague, which they contract from rats. They transmit tropical diseases such as typhus. They cause a plethora of minor problems such as itching and hives. However, the major cause of fleas in humans is more rudimentary: infestation from house pets, particularly dogs, which act as intermediary hosts for these pests.

Flea combat kit
- oil of oregano — burn the fleas out of the skin by applying the oil of oregano topically.
- oil of cumin — take 20 drops twice daily internally. Also, place on flea bites; they can't tolerate cumin.
- oil of bay leaf — highly valuable as a fumigant.
- oil of lavender — rub on involved regions and use for fumigation.

Note: pump spray the house with an oil of oregano and/or oil of bay leaf mixture. Use diffusers and atomizers; bomb them out with essential oils. It is curious to note that the medical treatment for flea infestation includes fumigation with mothballs (naphthalene), which is so poisonous that the house must be vacated for 48 hours. This is the beauty of using essential oils, which are actually therapeutic when burned or volatilized. Note: avoid all perfumes/colognes.

Flesh eating bacteria

No bacteria can digest human flesh by itself; but its enzymes can. This disease is not new. Known by the medical name *necrotizing fasciitis*, this disorder has been recognized as a common side effect of infection for over 50 years. The word necrotizing belies its ominous nature, because this is defined in medical dictionaries as "the mass death of human tissue (even bone)." The involved bacteria secrete potent enzymes capable of digesting any type of human protein, essentially liquifying anything in its path.

The high vulnerability of this infection in children may be due to the increasing use of certain drugs, which depress the immune system, making children more vulnerable to relentless infection. Researchers in Seattle found that children who consume anti-pain medication, particularly ibuprofen (Pediaprofen, etc.), are at a high risk for developing the infection.

This level of destruction can only be caused by bacteria capable of secreting potent enzymes. If produced in a sufficient amount, these enzymes can digest protein, including the protein of human skin, tissue, muscle, and bone. This is what happens in the flesh eating disease. The key is to destroy the germ and, thus, totally halt enzyme production. Another objective is to neutralize the existing bacterial enzymes and/or toxins responsible for the damage. Strep and staph, especially the drug resistant varieties, are the major progenitors of this disease. These germs are notoriously resistant to antibiotics, but they succumb to the powers of essential oils. What's more, natural plant enzymes can be consumed to neutralize the bacterial enzymes. Papain and bromelain are perhaps the most effective of these. These plant enzymes help denature, that is inactivate, the destructive bacterial enzymes.

Flesh eating bacteria combat kit
• raw honey — pack all over wounded area; also, eat 1/4 cup daily.
• oil of oregano (SuperStrength is best) — take 3 or more drops under the tongue as often as necessary, perhaps every few minutes. Also, take 5 to 10 drops in juice or water every hour or two. Important note: pour liberally on wound.
• Flavin-C — take 3 capsules every hour or two.
• oil of lavender (wild type) — add to wound and rub on surrounding skin, soles of feet, and buttocks.
• zinc chelate — take 100 mg daily until condition is resolved.
• premium-grade royal jelly (Royal Kick) — take 4 capsules several times daily.
• Oregamax capsules — take 3 or more capsules several times daily.
• Black seed-plus — take 3 capsules three times daily.
• uncoated bromelain plus papain (BromaZyme) — take 3 capsules several times daily.

Things to avoid
• refined sugar, soda pop, chocolate, and caffeine
• pain medications, especially aspirin and ibuprofen

Flu
Few people realize that influenza is the number one cause of death from infection in the United States. While other killers, such as Ebola, Hantavirus, and E. coli, seem to dominate the headlines,

they are insignificant as a cause of disability and death in comparison. For instance, while Hantavirus killed 60 and E. coli approximately 10 in 1993-94, the flu killed tens of thousands, some 60,000 in 1993 alone. A flu virus induced national crisis is completely plausible. In 1999 the flu struck certain regions in the United States with exceptional ferocity, the East Coast bearing the brunt of the damage. Essentially, the entire state of of Connecticut was disabled. Hospitals were overwhelmed, and admissions were halted. This was a modern-day medical catastrophe. Thus, the flu is the number one agent that must be derailed in the event of crisis. Of even greater consequence are the repercussions of hurricane Floyd: millions of dead animals floating in a stagnant infection soup. Included in these dead animals are the carcasses of some 100,000 pigs. It was Dr. J. Taubenburger of the Armed Forces Institute who reported in the *Associated Press* that the devastating 1918 flu was due to pig viruses, not from the Orient but from the United States. Thus, indirectly hurricane Floyd could induce a violent 1999-2000 flu epidemic, which could cause tens of thousands of fatalities.

The flu virus is a rather weak germ. It is highly vulnerable to natural antiseptics. A study performed by *Medical Science Research* determined that both RNA and DNA viruses were completely destroyed, that is the viruses were disentigrated, by oil of oregano. Use the wild high mountain type if possible, since this is the type which is proven by research to be the most powerful. Other anti-viral oils included oils of rosemary, bay leaf, cumin, and lavender. The virus destroying powers of raw garlic and onion are also well published. The raw forms are the most effective.

Flu combat kit
• oil of oregano (use SuperStrength for tougher cases) — take 2 drops under the tongue as often as possible, perhaps every few minutes. Also, take 5 to 10 drops three times daily in juice or water.
• Oregamax capsules — take 3 capsules three times daily.
• Flavin-C — take 2 or more capsules every few hours.
• Oil of Bay Berry — rub on face, neck, chest, and soles of feet.

Foods that help
• hot meat based broths with onion and garlic
• tangerine, grapefruit, and/or tomato juice

- anything high in vitamin A, like organic liver, salmon, sardines, etc.

Things to avoid
- chocolate and refined sugar (impede the immune response)
- soda pop and other sugary drinks as well as milk products

Food poisoning (see also individual illnesses)

Food poisoning develops when the individual consumes food or beverages which are either infected with or contaminated by microbes. It is the most common cause of sudden illness globally. Every day, hundreds of thousands of Americans contract food poisoning, largely from eating outside of the home. In other words, restaurant, catered, institutional, and picnic food is the source of the majority of cases of food related illness. The individual may become ill in the home, but this is much less common as a source of severe food borne illness compared to eating out.

According to the *Associated Press* when food poisoning outbreaks occur on a large scale there is no way to warn everyone. In one instance it was discovered early in the crisis that commercial ice cream was heavily contaminated with Salmonella. Despite the warnings aired on national TV several thousand individuals became ill. Thus, the government cannot completely protect the public in the event of an epidemic. Yet, protection can be found in wild spices, like oil of oregano and oil of cilantro/coriander, which pack enormous antiseptic powers.

No one is immune from this epidemic. Even healthy eaters and vegetarians are vulnerable. *Family Practice News* reports that organic vegetables, which were not carefully washed, caused an E. coli epidemic, which lead to the death of a child. A similar epidemic involving commercial red lettuce lead to the death of 25 people in Illinois. According to the CDC some 20,000 Americans were sickened from Salmonella/E. coli tainted alfalfa/radish sprouts in 1995 alone.

Bacteria are only one component of this crisis. The role played by parasites may be even greater. Parasites are larger organisms than bacteria, and include worms, flukes, amoebas, and protozoa. In the United States a wide range of parasites may be contracted from food, causing diarrheal diseases. Incredibly, one researcher described a rate of parasitic infections in U.S. citizens as high as 74%. The majority of these germs were likely contracted by eating contaminated food or drink. Foods commonly infested with parasites include raw meat, raw fish (sushi), vegetables, and fruit. To minimize the risks, be sure to carefully wash and/or peel all fruit and vegetables and avoid the consumption of raw meat.

Food poisoning combat kit
• oil of oregano — 2 or more drops under the tongue repeatedly until symptoms abate. Also, take 5 to 10 drops (or more) twice daily in juice or water.
• HerbSorb crushed Eastern herbal formula; take 2 capsules several times daily.
• Oregamax capsules — take 2 or more capsules several times daily or as much as is needed to halt the symptoms.
• raw honey — 1/4 cup two or three times daily.
• Lactobacillus — take several capsules daily.
• Oil of Cilantro/Coriander — add to food freely as needed.

Foods that help
• vinegar
• horseradish
• raw garlic
• cilantro/coriander (or Oil of Cilantro-plus)

Fractures
Little can be done by the lay person for this condition. It requires immediate medical care. Only rarely would the general public be called upon to assist in care. However, in the event that medical care is not accessible, utilize the following home remedies:

Fracture combat kit
• MCHC (microcrystaline hydroxyapatite or a high quality calcium chelate) — these forms of calcium may be unusually helpful in the process of rebuilding bone. Take 3000 mg daily for at least two weeks (this dose may be too much for individuals with a history of kidney stones). When taking this amount of calcium, be sure to drink plenty of water.
• bromelain/papain combination — take 3 capsules three or more

times daily on an empty stomach.

• oil of oregano — anti-pain, anti-inflammation. Take 10 drops three times daily. Rub topically as needed.

• Oregamax wild oregano capsules — rich in naturally occurring calcium and phosphorus, it provides nutrients for bone healing. Large amounts must be taken, like 12 capsules daily.

• Royal Kick — high grade royal jelly helps combat stress and speed healing.

• zinc — this nutrient speeds the healing of any wound; take at least 75 mg daily.

• silica — organically bound silica speeds the healing of bone injuries.

Note: Individuals with severe fractures must be kept still. If the individual must be moved, make a splint to immobilize the involved region as much as possible to prevent further damage.

Things to avoid
• caffeine and refined sugar, both of which deplete trace minerals
• diuretic drugs (also cause the urinary loss of minerals)

Frostbite

This is one of the most dangerous of all tissue injuries. It is caused by a sudden collapse of the small blood vessels which feed the skin and soft tissues. When the tissues are frozen by exposure to extreme cold, blood flow is curtailed and, thus, there is no oxygen delivery to the tissues. This leads to death of the involved tissues, known as gangrene.

Frostbite is largely preventable. Proper clothing is essential. The individual must realize that metal is the coldest substance, because it retains cold energy. Thus, touching cold metal with bare skin is one of the easiest ways to get frostbite.

Hot, tangy herbs/spices are highly protective against the cold, because they help the body produce and dissipate heat. Thus, the key to preventing and treating this condition is to accelerate the heat index of the blood. This is a novel concept, wherein the metabolic rate and blood flow are increased so that the body and the blood are highly resistant to cold. Certain trace minerals are particularly effective in accelerating metabolism, notably magnesium and potassium. Spices are top sources of these minerals. Plus, hot spices contain substances, notably the flavonoids and phenols, that accelerate blood flow. To protect yourself against the cold eat hot, spicy food.

Frostbite combat kit
• aloe vera — apply to the frostbite region; use it straight from the plant.
• oil of oregano — apply liberally as often as possible; also, take a few drops under the tongue often.
• oil of rosemary — apply to the frostbite region, and take 10 drops twice daily in juice or water.
• pantothenic acid — take 500 mg every few hours to help induce healing.
• raw honey — apply to the frostbite region.
• cayenne pepper — for prevention, add to shoes or inside gloves (the same can be accomplished with oil of oregano).
• Oil of Bay Berry — apply topically to speed wound healing.
• salt; add a half teaspoon in 12 ounces of water and sip (helps improve the pumping power of the heart, aiding blood flow).
• bromelain — take 4 capsules three or more times daily on an empty stomach.
• Juice of Sage and/or Essence of Orange Blossom — add to hot water and drink as a tea; drink several cups daily.

Foods that help
• *Taber's Medical Dictionary* advises to drink beef broth instead of pop or juice.
• plenty of hot herbal teas (sage tea is the best)

Things to avoid
• candy, sweets, and sugary drinks
• caffeine, chocolate, soda pop (caffeine and cocoa's theobromines impair circulation to the extremities)

Gallbladder attack

No one can imagine the dilemma of suffering a gallbladder attack without medical help. Yet, not every attack need result in gallbladder surgery.

Individuals with gallbladder problems are making a grave error by avoiding the consumption of fat. The gallbladder thrives on fat. Without it, the organ degenerates. As reported in *Medical Tribune,* March, 1993, low fat diets place individuals at "substantial risk of developing gallstones." The authors note that fat causes the gallbladder to "fully contract", in other words, it totally empties, which is the main way to prevent gallstones.

How to combat gallstones and gallbladder attacks:
• extra virgin olive oil — drink a quarter cup with a few tablespoons of vinegar two or three times daily; this should purge the gallbladder of stones and, thus, halt the attacks.
• oil of cumin — take 10 or more drops added into each olive oil purge (stimulates bile formation and aids in stone dissolution). Then, take 10 to 20 drops daily on a regular basis.
• oil of rosemary — take 10 or more drops twice daily (this may also be added to the olive oil purge or can be taken separately).
• HerbSorb — take 2 or more capsules with each meal.
• Nutri-Sense protein/lecithin drink mix (contains fatty acids and lecithin, which help dissolve stones) — take 3 heaping tablespoons in the morning in juice or water.
• oil of fennel (edible type in olive oil) — an important aid to gallbladder function, take 10 to 20 drops twice daily.

Foods that help
• avocados, Greek-style olives, and extra virgin olive oil
• vinegar
• fresh beef and/or lamb, fat included
• fresh calf's or lamb's liver, organic

Things to avoid
• eggs (in allergic individuals yolk may incite a gallbladder attack)
• white bread, white rice, refined sugar, sweets, soda pop
• fried food and/or margarine
• bakery items, sweet rolls, and/or cookies

Genital Herpes
It is estimated that a minimum of one fifth of all Americans suffer from this infection. In individuals under 30 years of age perhaps one of three have it. This may account for the recent estimation that as many as 50 million Americans harbor the germ. Thus, this viral infection is an epidemic of enormous proportions.

The herpes virus has a predilection for infecting the genitals, largely because of the rich supply of blood and nerves in this region. The virus may reside in blood vessels, within human cells, and in the nerves, while failing to cause obvious symptoms. The fact is the virus preferentially lives in the nerves, specifically the tiny condensations of nerve bodies known as *ganglia*. There are dozens of ganglia in the nerves of the pelvis buried deep in the low back, buttocks, sacral region, and inner pelvis. The virus hides there, only to resurface after traveling down the nerves to the skin and mucous membranes of the genitals as well as on the buttocks. The infection is incited by stress, cortisone intake, high amounts of chocolate/sugar, and vitamin deficiency. However, the most common cause is merely exposure: contracting the infection from an infected individual through sexual intercourse.

Genital herpes combat kit
• oil of oregano — dilute as follows: add 5 drops into a tablespoon of olive oil and apply directly to involved regions. Also, fill gelatin capsules and take 2 or 3 capsules twice daily.
• oil of myrtle — apply to involved region as often as necessary.
• Oregamax capsules — take 3 capsules twice daily.
• Black seed-plus (to stimulate immunity) — take 3 capsules twice daily.
• oil of cumin — take 10 drops twice daily in juice or water.

Things to avoid
• chocolate especially (the high arginine content of this food stimulates the growth of herpes viruses)
• nuts, especially peanuts (high in arginine)
• infected humans

Giardia and/or Cryptosporidium infection

This is already an epidemic. According to *American Family Physician,* February, 1998, in 1984 there were just six proven outbreaks of Giardia infection, i. e. giardiasis. In 1993-94 there were 34 outbreaks. In 1998 there were over 100. The infection usually occurs in the summer, but in children attending day care centers it may occur continuously.

Giardiasis is caused by a parasite, an organism larger and more difficult to kill than a bacteria. Contaminated water or contact with animal/human feces is the usual instigator. Campers and outdoors buffs frequently contract it from drinking untreated "natural" water from lakes and/or streams.

Giardia has a predilection for infecting the intestines, specifically the upper part of the duodenum. Thus, it may produce symptoms typical of a stomach ulcer. Symptoms of Giardia infection include:

- foul smelling sloppy stools
- diarrhea
- bloating
- flatulence, which is foul smelling (like rotten eggs)
- constant belching, especially in the morning
- nausea
- weight loss and lack of appetite

Giardia readily infests the gut, preferring the upper part of the small intestine and lower stomach. It may also infect the colon. The organism causes massive damage, leading to poor digestion and absorption. This is why weight loss, exhaustion, abnormal stools, and malabsorption of nutrients is so common in chronic Giardia infection.

Cryptosporidium, another water-based protozoan, causes a similar infection. The ultimate source is apparently sewage runoff from farm animals. This germ may aggressively attack the sick, weak, or immune compromised and may case death.

Giardia/Cryptosporidium combat kit

- oil of oregano — take 10 or more drops three times daily in juice or water.
- Oregamax — take 3 capsules twice daily.

- raw garlic — eat 2 or more cloves daily.
- Black seed-plus — take 3 or more capsules three times daily.
- BromaZyme — take 2 or more capsules twice daily on an empty stomach.

Head lice (see Lice)

Headaches

There are hundreds of causes for headaches. However, the major factors are food intolerance and hormonal disturbances, which, in all likelihood, many sufferers already suspect exist. These subjects are covered in great detail in my book, *Who Needs Headaches* (how to eliminate headaches and migraines without drugs). It is available by calling 1-800-243-5242. The ISBN number, which is useful when ordering it from the bookstore is 0911119329. Through this book you will learn in detail the main causes of headaches and how to address these causes through alternative medicine. The critical role of food allergies and hormonal disturbances in migraines is emphasized and explained.

Headache combat kit
- ginger root — slice the fresh root and immerse in hot water as a tea.
- Agonex capsules — special Native American herbal formula for this condition; take 2 capsules every hour to halt the attack. Take 2 capsules daily as a preventive.
- oil of oregano — rub on painful regions, forehead, temples, and/or sinus region. Take 1 or 2 drops under the tongue twice daily.
- oil of lavender — rub on forehead, chest, and soles of feet; take 2 drops under the tongue 3 or more times daily.
- Royal Kick premium royal jelly — to regenerate adrenal gland function, take 4 to 6 capsules every morning.
- Resvitanol (a must for its valuable arterial tonics) — chew on a teaspoonful to help stop the pain.

Things to avoid
- candy, chocolate, soda pop, sweet rolls/dough nuts, cookies
- wine and beer
- wheat, corn, malt, and citrus fruit

Heart attack

A heart attack in the field is very difficult to combat for the lay person. First, how does the individual who is observing the event know for sure it is a heart attack? True, there are instances where it is completely obvious. Yet, often even doctors may be confused by the symptoms and may mis-diagnose it as "indigestion" or "stress." Since stress is perhaps the main cause of heart attacks, remedies which combat stress, such as royal jelly and wild rosemary, are ideal.

There are certain telltale signs of heart attacks that hold true in 90% of the instances. An individual may have one or, usually, several of these signs. These signs/symptoms include:

• sudden episode of severe chest pain over heart on the left chest
• sudden severe pain in the jaw
• left sided chest pain which runs down the left arm
• nausea
• vague indigestion sensations, usually in the upper abdomen, that can't be relieved
• left shoulder pain
• occasionally, right sided chest pain
• pale complexion and cold sweat (clammy)

Obviously, if such symptoms develop, seek medical care immediately. If such care is unavailable, combat it with the following home remedies:

Heart attack combat kit
• oil of cilantro — 2 drops under the tongue every hour.
• fresh onion juice (from yellow onions) — take only a tablespoon at a time. Give every hour, if tolerated. Rub onion juice on the chest. Onion juice contains substances that help dissolve blood clots.
• oil of rosemary — take 5 to 10 drops twice daily.
• oil of oregano — take 2 drops under the tongue once or twice daily. Rub on chest and over heart reflexes as an aromatic rejuvenator.
• Oregamax capsules — take 3 or more capsules twice daily.
• Juice of Rosemary — take 2 ounces twice daily.
• Royal Kick premium royal jelly – take 2 to 4 capsules several times daily.

Things to avoid
- Fear: heart attack victims are tense and scared. Attempt to soothe them. Don't add to their fears.
- caffeine, colas, iced tea, and sugary juices
- wine or other alcoholic beverages

Heart failure
In this condition the heart is unable to pump blood fast enough to prevent it from backing up into the venous system. First the lungs fill up with fluid. Then, the fluids overflow into the remaining tissues. The individual becomes essentially waterlogged.

Heart failure combat kit
- raw honey — take as much as 1/2 cup three times daily.
- oil of cilantro plus coriander — take 10 to 20 drops twice daily.
- coenzyme Q-10 — take 200 mg daily.
- carnitine — take 2 to 3 grams daily.
- magnesium chelate — take 800 to 1000 mg daily.
- vitamin E — take 800 I.U. daily.
- HerbSorb — take 4 or more capsules three times daily.
- oil of oregano — take 2 or 3 drops under the tongue 3x daily.
- Juice of oregano – take one ounce twice daily.

Foods that help
- cooked beef hearts
- avocados, olives, extra virgin olive oil

Things to avoid
- caffeine, chocolate, refined sugar, and soda pop
- processed meats (i.e. those containing nitrates)

Heat exhaustion/stroke
Heat can destroy anyone. The young and old, healthy and strong all can be decimated by it.

Being exposed to an excess of summer heat can lead to a variety of illnesses. Usually, heat causes relatively minor discomforts such as dizziness, fainting, muscle cramps, swelling, sunburn, and exhaustion. However, in certain individuals the excess heat can kill.

Heat exhaustion is largely the result of heat induced sweating, which depletes the body of water and electrolytes. The loss of fluid and/or its evaporation from the skin disrupts the body's normal cooling mechanism, which is entirely dependent upon the volume of the body fluids. As a result, the body core temperature may rise suddenly. Fortunately, most individuals become noticeably sick and attempt to shelter themselves from the heat. Typical symptoms include dizziness, weakness, malaise, nausea, vomiting, rapid heart rate, and headache.

Some individuals don't sweat much even when exposed to extreme heat. In fact, the hotter their bodies become the less they sweat. This is a dangerous circumstance, because, without sweating, there is no way to dissipate heat. The heat becomes trapped within the body, leading to physical collapse and, in the extreme, heat exhaustion or stroke. Such heat vulnerable individuals suffer from a bizarre but common condition known as adrenal insufficiency. The fact is lack of sweating is a warning of adrenal failure.

Heatstroke is the more extreme version of heat exhaustion. It is always a medical emergency. The elderly and individuals with chronic disease are at the highest risk. When the body loses its ability to dissipate heat, the body temperature rises suddenly. Sweating virtually stops. Literally, the individuals boil to death. Often, such individuals collapse and nothing can seemingly be done to revive them.

If heatstroke develops, medical help must be summoned immediately. The objective is to reduce the body temperature through any means possible. If such help is unavailable, the following steps may prove lifesaving:
• get the individual out of the sun.
• fan the body aggressively.
• apply cool water, ice packs, wet sheets, etc. Cool water and the application of water cooled cloths is preferable to ice.
• if a shower can be accessed, spray the shower water in the finest mist possible over the individual at a temperature of about 60 degrees Fahrenheit.

Note: be aware that aggressive attempts to cool the individual may lead to further shock. To avoid this massage the body vigorously with essential oils, particularly the spine, legs, buttocks, and feet. However, remember, this is a medical emergency, so seek professional help urgently. Do not attempt to treat this condition on your own unless there is no other option.

Heat exhaustion combat kit
• Royal Kick premium grade royal jelly — take 4 capsules every hour or as necessary until the condition improves.
• red grape powder (Resvitanol) — take 4 capsules two or more times daily. Or, place the powder in the mouth and allow to melt.
• Flavin-C — 3 to 4 capsules immediately, then 1 or 2 capsules every hour with mineral water.
• oil of lavender — rub on face, spine, and chest.
• oil of sage or rosemary — rub on feet and spine.

Heatstroke combat kit
• oil of lavender — rub on spine, face, under nose, and chest.
• oil of sage — rub on soles of the feet and spine.
• oil of rosemary — rub over spine and adrenal reflex (mid lower back).
• Royal Kick (if the individual can swallow) — 2 or more capsules every hour with mineral water.
• red grape powder (Resvitanol) — 2 or more capsules every hour with mineral water. Or, place the powder in the mouth and allow to melt.
• Flavin-C — 4 capsules immediately, then 2 or more capsules every hour with mineral water.
• Hercules Strength caps — take 3 or more caps three times daily.

Foods that help
• sea salt (add a teaspoon of salt to 12 ounces of water and sip)
• watermelon, salted
• cucumbers
• radishes and turnips

Things to avoid
• completely avoid all sugar sweetened drinks and caffeinated beverages

Hemorrhoids

This is due to pressure on the delicate veins of the lower rectum. It is frequently caused by constipation, although infection and nutritional deficiency are often involved. Vitamin C, bioflavonoids, vitamin K, folic acid, and vitamin E are usually lacking. However, a lack of fiber is the greatest nutritional deficit. Remember, hemorrhoids are veins. Thus, substances which nourish the venous tissues are invaluable for preventing, as well as eradicating, this condition.

Hemorrhoid combat kit
• Nutri-Sense (as a source of soluble fiber and bowel softening lignins) — take 3 heaping tablespoons daily.
• Flavin-C (as a source of crude vitamin C and flavonoids) — take 3 capsules three times daily.
• vitamin E — take 400 to 800 I.U. daily.
• Oil of Bay Berry — apply topically for shrinkage.
• bromelain (as a natural antiinflammatory) — take 3 or more capsules twice daily on an empty stomach.
• oil of myrtle — apply this flavonoid rich oil directly on the hemorrhoids.
• Oregamax capsules — take 2 or 3 capsules three times daily.

Foods that help
• water; be sure to drink at least 6 large glasses daily
• papaya and kiwi
• tangerines, apricots, and blueberries

Things to avoid
• refined sugar, soda pop, and candy
• white flour, bread, and white rice

Hepatitis

This is defined as inflammation of the liver. It is a destructive inflammation, leading to the death of liver cells. If untreated, the liver tissues become scarred. This is known as cirrhosis.

There are dozens of causes for the inflammation. The main ones include alcohol excess, drug abuse, prescription drugs, non-prescription drugs, as well as a wide range of germs. Primarily, viruses are the causative germs, but a variety of parasites, as well as fungi and bacteria, may cause it.

Hepatitis, particularly the viral type, is currently an American, as well as global, epidemic. As many as a half million Americans are newly infected every year. It's virtually like a viral flu of the liver in terms of incidence as well as severity. Public health officials seem puzzled as to why so many Americans are developing hepatitis. It is not so complex. The hepatitis viruses and parasites are contracted through contamination, whether through blood, filth, secretions, or sexual contact. In other words, close contact with human fluids, excretions, or secretions is virtually a prerequisite for the development of this disease. Another possibility is if human waste contaminates food or water. This is an indirect means of contracting this dreaded disease. Yet, ultimately, it is human waste that is causing it.

Hundreds of outbreaks of hepatitis occur in the United States every year. Yet, frequently, the source is never determined.

There are perhaps a dozen or more strains of hepatitis, with new ones seemingly discovered yearly. Hepatitis A is perhaps the most commonly occurring type globally. Recently, in the United states outbreaks have been traced to imported frozen fruit, particularly strawberries from Mexico. Hepatitis C has attracted the most interest lately; the infection is an epidemic in America. It is a hidden infection, presenting initially with relatively mild symptoms and then smoldering within the body, causing prolonged infection and, therefore, tissue damage. The infection may have existed 5 to 10 years or longer before it is diagnosed. This may explain why there are as many as 5 million Americans infected with this virus. However, evidence of it may be discovered early, especially if it develops after blood transfusions, a major source for the infection. Yet, blood transfusions are not the only source. Recent evidence indicates that it is readily transmitted sexually and if an individual has the virus, there is a least a 15% chance of contracting it from such an individual. Eventually, it will probably be proven that sexual transmission is the main cause.

Hepatitis combat kit
• oil of oregano (SuperStrength may be necessary) — 2 or 3 drops under the tongue several times daily. Also, take 5 to 10 drops in juice or water twice daily.
• oil of cumin — take 10 to 20 drops twice daily in juice or water.
• oil of fennel — same as above.
• oil of cilantro plus coriander — take 10 or more drops daily.
• HerbSorb — take 3 or more capsules with every meal.
• BromaZyme (to aid in digestion and reduce inflammation) — take 2 or 3 capsules with meals.

Foods that help
• sardines and salmon
• artichokes and beets
• radishes and turnips (black or Russian radish is best)

Things to avoid
• alcohol and all drugs, herbal preparations, etc. containing it
• refined sugar, white flour, white rice
• prescription and non-prescription drugs of all types (except interferon)

Herbicide poisoning (see Pesticide/herbicide poisoning)

Herpes (see Cold sores, Genital herpes, Shingles)

High blood pressure attack
High blood pressure, known medically as hypertension, is a common disease, but only in Westernized countries. Diet is a major factor in the cause of this disease. In other words, what an individual eats and drinks is directly related to creating high blood pressure. While the role of diet is immense, the primary cause is a mere beverage: alcohol. In my clinic fully 40% of all high blood pressure patients were social, or, more rarely, heavy drinkers. Complete removal of the alcohol caused the blood pressure to normalize rapidly. Dietary causes, as well as stress, were the major factors in the remaining patients. In this regard the major cause was the excessive consumption of caffeinated soft drinks. Yet, contrary to popular belief, fat is not the major culprit in the diet: it is sugar.

High blood pressure combat kit
- oil of rosemary — take 10 to 20 drops twice daily. For extremely high blood pressure, take 20 drops three times daily or take 5 drops under the tongue every hour.
- oil of cilantro/coriander — take 10 drops twice daily.
- oil of lavender— rub on face and chest at night for relaxation. Add to atomizer or diffuser. Take 2 drops under the tongue twice daily.
- Agonex — a natural tonic for the kidneys, take 2 or 3 capsules twice daily. For severe attacks take 2 capsules every hour.
- red grape powder (Resvitanol) — take 4 capsules three times daily or more often if necessary. Resvitanol is entirely safe to take in large quantities. **Note:** oil of oregano is a strong tonic for the heart. If under doctors care for high blood pressure, seek a doctor's advice before using.

Foods that help
- sardines, salmon, halibut, and/or herring

Things to avoid
- alcohol: absolutely none should be consumed
- refined sugar and all sweets, particularly soda pop

Hip pain
Sudden hip pain in women over 50 may be an ominous sign. It may signal a fracture of the hip.

Hip pain usually results from injury. In women it may be caused by bone loss, that is osteoporosis. Hip pain may be caused by strain in the low back, which leads to a type of referred pain to the hip. In this instance the low back must also be treated. A strained knee may also induce hip pain.

Sudden severe hip pain, knee, or back pain may all warn of fractures, particularly in women over 40. Such fractures may occur without trauma. In other words, the bones simply crack.

Hip pain/fracture combat kit
• oil of oregano — take 5 to 10 drops two or three times daily in juice or water and take 2 or 3 drops under the tongue several times daily or to tolerance. Rub the oil on the involved region twice or more daily.
• hydroxyapatite (a special type of calcium which seals and reverses bone damage) — take several hundred mgs daily.
• vitamin D (as cod liver or halibut oil caps) — 6,000 I.U. daily
• Oregamax (as a source of crude natural calcium and magnesium) — take 9 or more capsules daily.
• red grape powder — take one teaspoon three times daily.

Things to avoid
• large amounts of aspirin, ibuprofen, or acetaminophen
• Don't sleep on the stomach or back; sleep on the side instead

Other ideas: an expert in structural therapy might help ease the pain, that is a well trained D. O., chiropractor, acupuncturist, or body worker.

Histoplasmosis
This is a fungal infection primarily of the lungs. However, the germ often attacks the entire body.

Histoplasmosis is the epidemic of river country. It should be called "river fever." That is because the mold thrives in areas of constant moisture and is exceptionally prolific in the Ohio and Mississippi river valleys, where moderate temperatures encourage its growth. It is also common in the middle South and Appalachian regions in areas like Kentucky, Virginia, West Virginia, and Tennessee. This is a soil fungus that thrives in moderate climates with lots of moisture. Regions wherein there are large congregations of birds and, therefore, large amounts of bird droppings are to be treated warily. This is because bird droppings greatly accelerate the fungus' growth. The primary signs and symptoms of histoplasmosis include fever of unknown cause (this fever may last for months), fatigue, low blood count, low white count, intestinal or stomach ulcers, and asthmatic symptoms.

Histoplasmosis combat kit
• oil of oregano — take 2 or 3 drops under the tongue several times daily. Also, take 5 to 10 drops in juice or water twice daily.
• wild oregano herb (Oregamax capsules) — take 3 or more capsules twice daily.
• oil of rosemary — take 2 or 3 drops under the tongue twice daily; rub on chest or add to diffuser. Also, take 5 to 10 drops twice daily.
• oil of bay leaf — take 5 to 10 drops twice daily; add to diffuser and volatilize.

Foods that help
• raw garlic and onion as well as green onions
• hot, tangy spicy soups

Things to avoid
• humidifiers and damp rooms
• refined sugar, sweets, chocolate
• wheat or other common grains (they are often mold contaminated)

Hives
This reddish skin lesion is far from an illness of the skin. Allergic toxicity is the primary cause of hives. Foods, chemicals, drugs, food additives, and perfumes all may induce hives. They may also be caused by infections. Here, the primary culprits are parasites. Yet, even in this instance the parasites produce noxious chemicals, which provoke the hives.

Hives are usually signified by bright red blotches occurring virtually anywhere on the body. They represent an abrupt inflammation in the small blood vessels that supply the skin. The redness represents the extensive degree of inflammation and irritation which develops. It is obviously a toxic reaction to some substance, and this substance is usually something which is ingested, in other words, what we eat, breath, and drink causes the majority of cases of hives. Infection represents the second major cause, and parasites, as well as fungi, are the primary players. Insect bites may also result in hives. However, drug reactions are the number one cause; this is even more important as a cause than food.

Hives combat kit
- oil of oregano — use topically and internally, take liberally under the tongue and/or internally until lesions clear.
- wild oregano herb — either as Oregamax or Hercules Strength (the latter is useful in the event of allergy to onion or garlic); take 3 capsules three times daily.
- Royal Kick premium grade royal jelly (unless allergic to bee stings) — take 4 capsules every hour or two until condition clears.
- tea tree oil — apply topically only.
- red grape powder — take 4 capsules twice daily.

Things to avoid
- citrus fruit, particularly oranges, lemons, and limes
- wheat, rye, corn, and barley
- chocolate
- apple juice

Hookworm

According to Peters and Gilles, authors of *A Colour Atlas of Tropical Medicine and Parasitology*, fully a quarter of the world's population, billions of individuals, are infected with hookworms. This is astonishing, since this parasite can only thrive in hot climates. However, much of the global population is concentrated in tropical and subtropical regions, where hookworm infestation is endemic. Likely countries/regions in which the infection is contracted include India, Southern China, Malaysia, Indonesia, Northeastern Australia, Japan, Southeast Asia, Italy, Sicily, Northern Turkey, Egypt/North Africa, and Burma. In the Americas the parasite is found in the soil of virtually all of South America (except Chili and Argentina) and most of Central America. However, travelers to these regions are also vulnerable. They may contract the infection, which leads to chronic health problems, such as digestive disorders, fatigue, heart disease, weight loss, and skin diseases. In the United States hookworm infests primarily the Southeast, notably Florida, the Carolinas, Georgia, Louisiana, Alabama, Mississippi, Tennessee, Arkansas, Missouri, and parts of Texas. However, there is a complicating factor that has led to more widespread infestation in the United States: dog hookworm. This worm is disseminated primarily by dog feces. It may or may not cause systemic disease. Often, infection is represented by localized creeping tracts usually on the feet. Symptoms of systemic hookworm infection include:

- exhaustion
- weak muscles
- shortness of breath
- swelling in the extremities
- swollen abdomen
- vague digestive problems

Hookworm destruction/combat kit

- oil of oregano — take 10 or more drops three times daily in juice or water or Oreganol gelcaps, 3 or more caps daily.
- oil of cumin — take 10 drops three times daily in juice or water.
- oil of cilantro/coriander — take 10 drops three times daily in juice or water.
- oil of fennel — the top anti-hookworm oil, take 10 to 20 drops twice daily.
- raw garlic — eat as many cloves as possible.

Foods that help

- spinach and watercress (wash well)
- papaya and kiwi (always eat the papaya seeds)
- fresh red meat (cooked at least medium, to replenish parasite depleted blood)

Things to avoid

- raw meat or fish
- dog feces

Hot flashes

Hot flashes are regarded exclusively as a female problem. Now men are also suffering from them. The causes in men are unknown, although, like women, it is probably hormonal. In women the flashes are induced by an imbalance in hormone production. Specifically, it is believed that as women age, they fail to produce sufficient amounts of estrogens, resulting in a wide range of symptoms, including hot flashes, fatigue, mood swings, loss of libido, and depression.

Hot flashes combat kit
• royal jelly — 4 capsules every morning or Royal oil, 1-2 t.
• sage tea or oil of sage (edible type in olive oil) — drink the tea twice daily. Rub the oil on the mid-lower back (adrenal reflex).
• oil of fennel — 10 drops twice daily in juice or water.
• Essence of Orange Blossom (or white coffee) — add one or two tablespoons in hot water as a tea, preferably at night after supper. Also, add to cold drinks if desired.
• Hercules Strength — rosemary/sage herbal; take 2 or more capsules twice daily.
• oil of myrtle (for improving sex drive and reversing vaginal dryness) — rub on vaginal tissue twice daily.

Things to avoid
• chocolate and refined sugar
• synthetic estrogens

Hypothermia (see Cold exposure)

Impetigo

This is perhaps the most contagious of all childhood bacterial infections. It is usually caused by staph or strep; in some instances, both of these germs are involved.

Usually, impetigo strikes the face, notably the cheeks and especially around the mouth and nose. When it develops about the mouth and nose, it is often confused with cold sores (i.e. Herpes virus). It may also occur on the arms or legs. Typically, lesions form a pustule, which breaks, dumping germs. The germs readily spread and the contagion may strike anywhere on the body as well as infecting other individuals. To avoid the rampant spread of this infection do not touch the skin or pustules with bare hands. If any lesions are touched, wash hands thoroughly with soap and hot water; add a few drops of oil of oregano to pump or bar soaps to aid in antisepsis.

Impetigo combat kit
• oil of oregano (the most important herbal therapy) — apply topically and take internally.
• raw honey — apply topically
• Oregamax capsules — take 2 capsules every four hours.
• Oil of Bay Berry — apply topically to speed healing and minimize scarring

Things to avoid
• don't allow children to keep long fingernails. The impetigo germs may be housed underneath them. Keep the fingernails clipped.

Influenza (see Flu)

Ingrown toenail
This seems like a minor problem. Yet, an ingrown toenail can become extremely painful and can also result in secondary infection. It is usually caused when the individual is too aggressive with clipping of the toenail. Always clip the nail in a straight line. Don't clip the corners aggressively, because, if you do, the nail may grow into the skin, causing severe pain, inflammation, and infection.

Ingrown toenail combat kit
• oil of oregano — this is usually all you need; apply twice daily

Insecticide poisoning (see pesticide/herbicide poisoning)

Insomnia

During a crisis it is essential for the individual to rest. Lack of sleep quickly devastates human health during adversity. A rested body and mind provide the strength necessary to survive.

Insomnia is frequently related to blood sugar disorders. When the blood sugar drops, the brain misfires, leading to an irritated state. High protein snacks eaten late at night balance the blood sugar mechanism. To help relax the nervous system use sedative essential oils such as oils of sage, oregano, and lavender.

Insomnia combat kit
• oil of oregano — rub on chest and neck at bedtime.
• Juice of Sage — add two tablespoons in hot water and drink as a late night tea.
• calcium — take 1000 mg of a fine absorbable calcium at bedtime.
• oil of lavender — rub on chest and neck at bedtime. Add to a diffuser or atomizer.
• oil of sage — take a few drops in hot water or rub on feet or back.
• wild strawberry leaves and borage flowers (a natural sedative) — drink a cup of hot WildPower Tea before bedtime.

Foods that help
• salted roasted nuts, especially if eaten at bedtime
• salted turkey meat (sugar free), eat at bedtime
• full fat cheese, eat at bedtime

Itchy skin/scalp (see also Hives)

There are four common causes of itchy skin: contact with poisonous plants, allergic reactions to drugs or other chemicals, allergic reactions to foods, and fungal infections. Thus, the cause should be relatively easy to determine. Fungal infections may result in itchy skin, because fungi secreting poisons, which cause inflammation and, therefore, itching.

Itchy skin/scalp combat kit
• oil of oregano — this is the mainstay; rub on any itchy region.

Also, take 2 drops under the tongue as often as necessary.
Note: fungal organisms, like Candida albicans and tinea, can cause itchy skin by secreting poisons, which cause inflammation and therefore itching. Oil of oregano is antifungal.

• tea tree oil — use as needed, topically only.
• Oil of Bay Berry (a tremendous emollient for sensitive or itchy skin) — take 2 drops under the tongue three or more times daily.
• oil of myrtle — soothing for topically application; especially useful for itchy vaginitis.
• Might at Night™ — special essential oil formula for the scalp; rub solution into scalp and leave overnight, then shampoo with WHAMPOO in the morning.

Foods that help
• beets and beet juice (include beet tops, if possible)
• radishes, especially Russian or black radishes
• olive oil and vinegar (stimulates the flow of bile)

Things to avoid
• all drugs, including antihistamines and antibiotics
• alcohol of all types, including the use of alcohol as a base material
• lye based soaps and perfumes
• refined sugar (increases the growth of fungi)
• jewelry containing nickel

Jaundice
This is caused by liver damage. The damage is induced primarily by toxic chemicals and/or germs. Major causes of jaundice include alcohol abuse, drug abuse, prescription drug reactions, and viral hepatitis. The condition is manifested by the accumulation of bile pigments, i.e. bilirubin, in the skin as well as the whites of the eyes. Severe jaundice is an indication of massive liver damage.

Jaundice combat kit
• oil of cumin (a potent antioxidant for the liver) take 20 drops twice daily in juice or water.
• oil of rosemary (purges the liver of poisons and bile) — take the same as above.

- LivaClenz (a multi-edible essential oil formula for regenerating liver function and increasing glutathione synthesis) — take 10 or more drops three times daily.
- beet juice tablets or powder — take several tablets or a teaspoon three times daily.
- oil of oregano (especially valuable in the event of infection) — take 5 drops twice daily.

Foods that help
- beets and beet tops, ideally gently cooked
- radishes of all types, especially black/Russian radish

Jock itch (see Athlete's foot)

Joint pain
Joint pain may be a manifestation of a severe disease, or it may be due to injury. It may also warn of infection. This is especially true when it afflicts one joint only. Bacterial infection often causes pain in an isolated joint. However, parasitic infestation, particularly by amoebas, may cause pain in multiple joints. For instance, rheumatoid arthritis is believed to be due to a systemic amoebic infection. Single joint pain, like knee pain, may also warn of Lyme disease.

Joint pain combat kit
- oil of oregano — rub on involved region; take 2 or more drops under the tongue twice daily. Also, take 5 to 10 drops in juice or water twice daily.
- oil of rosemary — take 5 to 10 drops twice daily in juice or water.
- red grape powder — take 4 capsules twice daily (if using bulk, take a teaspoon or more daily).

Kidney infection
This is usually caused by bacterial infection, although yeast and parasitic infections are increasingly involved. These infections are particularly common in young children, especially girls. The elderly are also highly vulnerable. Kidney infections frequently

develop a consequence of prolonged surgeries, which require the placement of urinary catheters. The yeast Candida albicans is the most notorious culprit in post surgical kidney infections. Kidney infections which fail to improve despite repeated antibiotic therapy are likely due to yeast infestation. The yeasts thrive in the kidneys and may provoke repeated bladder infections; they may also cause bladder and vaginal yeast infections. The health dramatically improves when the kidneys are sterilized of all invaders.

Kidney infection combat kit
• oil of oregano — take 3 drops under the tongue three times daily. Also, take 10 to 20 drops in juice or water three times daily.
• red grape powder (Resvitanol) — take 4 capsules three times daily. For severe infections double this amount (for bulk consumption, take three or more heaping teaspoons daily. This is safe to take in large amounts, because it is a food like substance.
• oil of fennel (helps stimulate normal urine flow) — take 10 drops three times daily.
• WildPower Tea (natural diuretic for aiding stronger urination) — drink 2 or more cups daily.

Foods that help
• cranberry as a juice or extract — take often, as much as desired.
• Pomegranate Syrup — add a T. to water and drink twice daily.

Kidney stones
This is a disaster of major significance no matter what the circumstances. The pain of kidney stones is one of the most gruesome of all types of organ pain.

Repeated kidney stones are a sign of chronic infection. When germs infect the kidneys, they cause inflammation, and this leads to stone formation. The usual culprits are bacteria and fungi. Nutritional deficiency is another major factor. A lack of magnesium, potassium, pyridoxine, vitamin C, and even calcium may play a role. Vitamin D deficiency is also a factor, since this substance controls calcium metabolism and most stones are made of calcium. However, vitamin A deficiency is the primary factor inducing kidney stones. Chronic kidney stone formation nearly always warns of a severe vitamin A deficiency.

Kidney stones combat kit
• red grape powder (Resvitanol) — take 4 capsules three times daily.
• oil of fennel — take 20 drops three times daily.
• Oregamax capsules — take 6 or more capsules daily.
• magnesium and/or potassium citrate — take 1000 mg daily.
• Flavin-C — take 6 or more capsules daily.

Foods that help
• Pomegranate Syrup — mix a tablespoon in water and drink twice daily.
• organic calf's or lamb's liver (as a source of vitamin A) — eat a pound per week.
• cranberry (either concentrate or extract) — use as much as possible.
• parsley — chew on a bunch daily; or, make parsley juice and drink a cup daily.

Things to avoid
• caffeine, alcohol, chocolate
• refined sugar and all sweets
• calcium supplements made from oyster shell, calcium carbonate, dolomite, or bone meal

Killer bees (see also Bee stings)
A laboratory freak, killer bees are the scientist's worst nightmare. Now they have become a public menace of enormous proportions.

Killer bees are a product of genetic experiments in Brazil, an attempt by scientists to increase the productivity of local bees. They mated the placid local honey bees with aggressive African honey bees. The bees escaped from the lab and mated with Brazilian bees in the wild, corrupting their gene pool. These "synthetic" bees retained their aggressive nature and have become international monsters.

In only a few years the bees have hewn a path from Brazil

all the way to the Southern United States. They are now found in virtually all Southern states. In the process the bees have attacked hundreds of thousands of mammals, including humans, killing and maiming thousands. In fact, thousands of humans have been viciously attacked by killer bees, many fatally. Deaths from killer bees occur daily. The number of the human victims and the death and devastation they wreak is mounting. For those who proclaim that genetic engineering is for the benefit of humankind, here is merely one example of the devastation resulting from such human bungling and arrogance.

Killer bee combat kit
• oil of oregano (SuperStrength may be necessary) — rub this on any sting immediately. Also, drip it on the bees if they are attached. During the attack attempt to give several drops under the tongue frequently. Or, just get it into the mouth. If possible, find a pump spray bottle; add hot water and oil of oregano; spray the bees. Also, spray at any attacking bees. This will drive them off and/or kill them. The oil destroys their sensitive scent glands. Other anti-bee oils include oil of cumin, bay leaf, and, perhaps, tea tree oil.
• Oregamax capsules — give as many as possible.
• red grape powder (Resvitanol) — take as much as possible.
• pantothenic acid (500 mg capsules) — take 2 every hour to block circulatory shock.
Special Note: the key is to take the anti-toxic essential oils under the tongue for quick absorption into the blood. This is a life-saving maneuver. Give 2 or more drops of oil of oregano under the tongue repeatedly to halt or prevent shock related death. It is the shock, that is the collapse of the circulatory system that kills, not the bites by themselves.

Foods that help
• vinegar — pour full strength on bees and stings
• sea salt — drink a solution of salt water to block circulatory shock

Things to avoid
• perfumes

Laryngitis

Extreme hoarseness is the well known symptom of this condition, and people who have it commonly are reduced to a whisper or perhaps no voice at all. It is usually due to a virus, which can directly infect the vocal cords. The nerves to the vocal cords may also be subjected to attack. Laryngitis is usually induced by stress. It may also develop as a consequence of sinus infection, in other words, the infection begins in the sinuses and eventually induces the laryngitis. It is important to note that hoarseness may also be a warning of vocal cord cancer.

Loud speech, stress, or arguing may precipitate this condition. Constant consumption of allergenic foods also increases the risks.

Laryngitis combat kit
• oil of oregano — take 2 drops under the tongue every few hours or more often if necessary.
• oil of rosemary — take 10 drops twice or more daily.
• oil of sage — take 5 drops twice daily.
• Essence of Orange Blossom — highly soothing; add one or two tablespoons in warm water as a tea, adding raw honey if desired.
• raw crude honey — add to hot herbal tea or White Coffee and drink several times daily.

Foods that help
• Pomegranate Syrup — add a tablespoon to hot water and drink several times daily.
• raw honey or carob molasses — soothing and easy to consume

Things to avoid
• arguments
• chocolate (stimulates the growth of viruses)
• corn, wheat, and rye

Lead poisoning

Lead poisoning usually develops over a prolonged period. The vast majority of cases occur in individuals who work in factories which utilize lead. People living in in older homes which have old or lead paint. Regarding the latter the source is lead paint, lead containing dust, and lead water pipes.

Despite its well known toxic effects, American industry still relies upon lead. In fact, besides iron and steel lead is the most widely used industrial metal. This puts both workers and those living near the factories at risk. At the greatest risk include those in the following industries:

- battery
- construction
- demolition
- firing range
- foundry
- gas station
- jewelry
- pipe fitters/plumbers
- pottery
- soldering
- stained glass
- welding

Lead is absorbed through the skin, but ingestion or inhalation of lead particles are the major means of contamination. What's more, once entering the body lead is highly soluble in fatty tissues, so it readily pollutes the fatty brain, nerve sheaths, and spinal cord. Also, because it dissolves so easily into the tissues, it is difficult to remove. This heavy metal is also readily absorbed by bone, which binds it fiercely. This may account for the musculoskeletal symptoms so common in lead poisoning. Because of the fact that inhalation is a major means of lead contamination, wearing a mask is a simple and effective method to prevent lead exposure in the event of a major urban disaster. Early signs of lead poisoning include:

- fatigue
- memory loss
- irritability
- vague muscle, bone, or joint pain
- headaches
- stomachaches and cramps
- numbness

As the illness progresses the following symptoms may develop:

- impotence and/or loss of sex drive
- vague digestive problems
- loss of sensation in arms/legs
- weight loss
- constipation
- vomiting
- constant headache

Chronic lead poisoning also results in anemia. Thus, in an individual suffering from these symptoms who is also anemic, lead poisoning is virtually assured.
Sudden exposure to lead exhibits certain symptoms, notably:
- abdominal tightness, cramps, and colic
- constipation
- severe fatigue
- convulsions, vomiting, seizures, and other symptoms of brain damage

Sudden overwhelming lead exposure could occur during a disaster, especially earthquakes or toxic chemical releases. Chelation therapy is the only way to extract large amounts of lead. This is the irreversibly binding of the metal so that it can be eliminated through the kidneys and gut. Medically, this requires a type of intravenous therapy. It involves the IV infusion of a drug called EDTA, which binds, that is chelates, the lead and removes it from the body through the kidneys. However, this is impractical during a crisis. The following is a protocol of natural substances which bind and remove lead from the body:

Lead poisoning detoxification kit
- oil of cumin and coriander (to purge the liver of bile and lead molecules) — take 20 drops of each twice daily.
- oil of rosemary — take 20 drops twice daily.
- calcium chelate (helps drive lead out of bone) — take 2000 mg daily.
- Oregamax capsules — a major aid for chelating heavy metals, take 4 capsules three times daily.
- red grape powder (Resvitanol) — rich in organic acids, which

aggressively bind heavy metals, take 4 or more capsules three times daily. If using bulk, take 3 or more teaspoons daily.
• magnesium chelate — take 800 mg daily (do not use magnesium oxide).

Things to avoid
• all calcium supplements made from bone meal and oyster shell calcium (high in lead residues)

Leg cramps
This is almost exclusively due to nutritional deficiency. Poor circulation may also play a role. Nutrients which are primarily deficient include pantothenic acid, folic acid, calcium, magnesium, sodium, potassium, and vitamin E.

Calcium deficiency may be the major factor in the cause of leg cramps in women, particularly in those who shun the typical calcium rich foods such as fresh milk, cheese, yogurt, sardines, canned salmon, and dark greens. What's more, since calcium absorption is dependent upon vitamin D, leg cramps may also warn of a deficiency of this sunshine dependent nutrient. This may also explain why some women have an increase in leg or foot cramps during the winter. Liver disease increases the risks for leg cramps, because the liver produces a protein required for calcium transport.

For immediate relief rely on antiinflammatory essential oils. Rub these oils over the involved region to enhance blood flow and reduce pain and relax the nervous system.

Leg/foot cramp combat kit
• pantothenic acid — take 500 mg twice daily.
• vitamin E — take 800 to 1200 I.U. daily.
• oil of lavender — rub on involved region.
• oil of oregano — rub on involved region and take 2 drops under the tongue repeatedly until cramps stop.
• oil of rosemary — take 5 drops under the tongue repeatedly until cramps stop.
• folic acid — take 5 to 10 mg daily.

• calcium and magnesium — take 2000 mg of calcium and 800 mg of magnesium daily.
• Royal Kick (an excellent source of natural pantothenic acid; aids cortisone production) — take 4 capsules twice daily.

Foods that help
• glass of warm milk with honey (the natural sugars in the honey aid in calcium absorption)
• large handful of salted almonds, filberts, or roasted peanuts

Lice
Having lice crawling on the body or in the hair elicits all manner of emotional reactions. The thought alone can create hysteria. The most common type is the one which attacks the hair and scalp, i.e. head lice. Other types include body lice, and pubic lice.

Head lice attack the scalp, because it is a warm climate, perfect for their metabolism. Obviously, bald individuals are innately protected. The lice tend to adhere close to the scalp, because they require body heat to survive. The eggs are also found close to the scalp and are attached to the hair follicles. The main site for egg attachment is the back of the head. The problem is that the infection festers without symptoms for perhaps weeks before it is discovered. By then the entire family and home may become infested.

Essential oils are the remedy of choice. Their solvent action makes them ideal for combating this condition, because the oils dissolve the eggs. Plus, the antiseptic powers of the oils kill the live lice outright. To begin treatment, comb repeatedly with a metal or hard plastic comb; start combing from the base of the scalp forward. If possible, saturate the comb with anti-lice essential oils such as oil of bay, fennel, cumin, or oregano. Cover the entire head twice or more daily from the back of the scalp to the front.

Lice combat kit
• oils of oregano, fennel, cumin, and bay leaf: add one part of each oil together; rub into scalp and hair. Repeat as often as necessary until all lice and eggs are destroyed. Or, use Might at Night™.

• oil of oregano: take 2 or 3 drops under the tongue twice daily.
• diffuser or atomizer: fumigate the rooms with oils of oregano, lavender, fennel, and/or bay leaf.
• metal comb and wash hair with Whampoo (with essential oil blasting power)
Note: Might at Night has recently become available. It contains a combination of aromatic essential oils. While not marketed as anti-lice, it contains cumin, oregano, fennel, etc. in one formula. It is safe, because the oils are natural and edible. Simply rub the formula into the hair as often as possible and/or on the body as needed. It is also a tremendously valuable natural hair conditioner. Remember, mites, lice, fungi, and bacteria all can inhabit the hair and scalp. To order Might at Night and Whampoo call 800-243-5242.

Lyme disease

Lyme disease is caused by the bite of ticks, usually the so called deer ticks. This disease is an epidemic in the East Coast, however, cases have been reported virtually everywhere. Regions at the highest risk include New York and New Jersey,

Lyme is supposedly one of the most difficult to diagnose of all diseases. Yet, it shouldn't be. Lyme mimics the flu, that is it is represented by mild to moderate muscle aches, fever, malaise, etc. Yet, the flu rarely occurs in the spring and summer, which is when Lyme usually strikes. A significant percentage of Lyme victims develop a rash a week or so after the tick bite. The rash is non-itching and circular. No such rash is seen in the flu.

It is a major error to mis-diagnose Lyme disease as the flu. This is because a large percentage of infected individuals develop chronic disease, which may be debilitating or even life threatening. Great effort must be made to procure a precise diagnosis. High suspicion should exist for wilderness buffs, who develop sudden flu-like illnesses during the spring or summer. Dog owners are also a high risk category, especially if the dogs venture outdoors. Erroneous diagnosis and/or treatment may result in chronic Lyme, which is devastating. Symptoms of chronic Lyme include joint pain, stiff spine or neck, muscle aches, exhaustion, poor concentration, headaches, numbness, and fatigue.

Lyme is difficult to cure by any means, medical or herbal. However, recent data indicates that prolonged treatment of the individual with anti-Borrelia compounds, whether natural or synthetic, offers hope for a cure. For instance, researchers, publishing in *Modern Medicine*, September, 1997, determined that after a 90 day course of tetracycline over 60% of Lyme patients improved significantly. However, it is important to note that long term antibiotic therapy has numerous risks, for instance the development of fungal infections as well as drug resistant mutants. This is why natural substances are so valuable. There is no risk with long term use of natural substances with germ killing power such as cinnamon, oregano, garlic, cumin, onion, etc. Rather, there is often significant improvement, perhaps cure. At a minimum medicine along with natural cures should be combined to provide the individual with the best odds for a cure.

Medical authorities have deluded themselves to believe that a tick bite leads to only one circumscribed infection. Ticks are fully contaminated with a wide range of germs, which they derive from the blood of rodents. Thus, usually, multiple infestations result from a single bite. This is clearly evidenced by an article published by researchers at the University of Wisconsin; these researchers discovered that a significant percentage of Lyme patients also had in their blood other tick-acquired germs. It is likely that perhaps dozens of different germs are injected by a single tick bite. Recall that Lyme smoldered in humans in this country for decades before it was discovered. This illustrates the importance of natural antiseptics, such as oil of oregano, which are capable of attacking a wide range of invaders. Bombard these germs from your body with every tool possible.

Tick combat kit (for destroying the tick)
• fine point straight tweezers
• oil of oregano (SuperStrength is best) — saturate a cotton ball and hold over tick until it dies. Remove the dead tick carefully with tweezers. Grab the tick as close to its attachment as possible.
• tea tree oil — also useful by saturating tick or a cotton ball held over it.

• oil of bay leaf — also for pouring on the tick or cotton ball.
• cotton balls (saturate with the oils and suffocate the tick)

Tick disease combat kit (in case of infection)
• oil of oregano (Superstrength is preferable) — take 2 or more drops under the tongue three times daily. Also, take 10 to 20 drops in juice or water twice daily. For extremely tough conditions, double this amount. Oreganol capsules are an alternative, 2 or more daily.
• oil of cumin — take 10 drops twice daily in juice or water.
• wild oregano herb (Oregamax capsules) — take 3 capsules three times daily.
• red grape powder (Resvitanol) — take 4 capsules three times daily.
• Juice of Oregano — take one or more ounces twice daily.

Foods that help
• papaya and its seeds
• horseradish
• raw garlic and onion; also, onion/radish juice

What to do if a tick is attached

• Don't touch the tick with your hands unless no other option is available.
• Saturate the tick with oil of oregano and/or tea tree oil.
• Saturate a cotton ball with these oils and hold the ball gently over the tick. Do this until the tick suffocates (dies).
• When dead, grasp the tick as close as possible to its attachment site with the tweezers. Pull the tick out slowly but gently. If the tick is crushed and secretions pour out, saturate the involved region with tea tree or oregano oil and wash the region, as well as the hands, thoroughly.
• If tweezers are unavailable, cover the fingers with tissue or a paper towel (or a plant leaf) and pull out the tick. Do not cut the tick open, as this will spread its dangerous secretions and blood. Kill it with the essential oils.

How to Avoid Tick Bites

If you are in a tick infested region and are exposed to the elements, here are some simple steps that may help protect you:

• Never sit directly on the ground, and avoid sitting or squatting near tall grass.
• If you must sit on the ground, place light colored sheets or bedding underneath you. Or, place cardboard or plywood on the ground. This will make it easier to see ticks.
• Wear socks over the pants to force ticks to crawl up the legs so they can be spotted.
• Tuck shirts into pants and wear tight long sleeve shirts, if possible.
• Take the time to inspect for ticks regularly, no matter how time consuming or difficult it seems.
• DEET containing tick repellents are potentially carcinogenic. If possible, use natural tick repellents. However, it may be necessary to maintain a can or two of commercial tick repellent in case all else fails. Premethrin is a less toxic alternative to DEET. However, this is applied to the clothing rather than the skin. One application lasts about two weeks to keep the ticks away.

Malaria

Once exclusively a tropical disease, malaria has invaded temperate regions: through travelers. This does not mean that outbreaks will occur in Chicago or New York city. Yet, it is remotely possible that pockets of infection could develop in the Southern United States.

There is an effective drug for malaria, a quinine derivative, yet, it is not without side effects. Still, the condition is highly serious and relying upon drug therapy alone may be inadequate.

The fact is this germ is difficult to kill, because it hides inside red blood cells. It does so to evade the immune system, plus it feeds upon these cells. The malaria parasite should be bombarded with every possible antiseptic/antiparasitic substance available.

Malaria combat kit
• oil of oregano (SuperStrength is best) — take 2 or more drops under the tongue several times daily. Also, 10 to 20 drops in juice or water twice or more daily or use Oreganol caps (one cap equals 7 drops of oil).
• wild oregano capsules (Oregamax) — take 6 or more capsules
• oil of cumin — 5 or more drops twice daily
• Juice of Oregano — 2 ounces twice daily

Measles (regular and German)
This is highly contagious, perhaps one of the most contagious infections known. Measles begins with a cough, high fever, eye irritation, with the development of a rash within 4-5 days. Ear infections, as well as viral pneumonia, may develop afterwards. Rarely, if the fever is high enough and if the child becomes severely dehydrated, brain damage may occur.

German measles is also known as "3 day measles." Less contagious and harsh, it is only a threat in pregnant women, who may pass the infection to the fetus. Birth defects are believed to be a possible consequence. Symptoms are a rash, fever, fatigue, and aching limbs. The following amounts are appropriate for children.

Measles combat kit
• oil of oregano — take 2 drops under the tongue twice daily; also, take 2 drops in juice or water twice daily. Add to raw honey.
• Oregamax capsules — take 3 or more capsules daily.
• Oil of Bay Berry — rub on any rash, also on the buttocks, soles of feet, and chest.
• oil of wild lavender — add to diffuser and rub on the body.
• Flavin-C — take 2 capsules three times daily.

Things to avoid
• soda pop; give juice instead (this at least provides vitamin C)
• chocolate, beans, nuts, and seeds

Melanoma

In California medical scientists list melanoma as an absolute epidemic. It has risen in incidence at a stupendous rate throughout the United States. In 1935 the individual had only a 1 in 2000 risk of developing it. Now the risk is nearly 1 in 75. That is an epidemic.

Melanoma may develop anywhere on the body and can even occur in the mouth and under the nails. However, it most commonly occurs on the torso, oddly enough, in areas not regularly exposed to the sun. This is supposedly a sun-induced disease. Yet, its distribution certainly gives credence to the theory that regular measured exposure to the sun is somehow protective. In fact, a study in Canada of thousands of men regularly exposed to the sun as outdoor workers showed a decreased incidence of melanoma compared to the normal work force.

When this disease strikes, it elicits great fear. There is no need to fear. As always, medical treatment should ideally be combined with nutritional support. Certain vitamin deficiencies are associated with heightened melanoma risk and these nutrients should be supplemented in the diet. A lack of vitamins A, C, E, D, and beta carotene all increase the risk for melanoma. These nutrients should be taken to prevent it as well as to eradicate it after it strikes. B vitamins which protect against it include pyridoxine and riboflavin. Selenium and zinc also offer protection. As always, be sure to seek medical care if a suspicious lesion develops.

Melanoma Combat Kit

- wear white/light colored cotton clothing that covers most of the exposed parts
- large brimmed hats are mandatory
- top quality sunscreen containing antioxidants
- oil of oregano — rub into the lesion three times daily. Also, take 2 or 3 drops under the tongue twice daily.
- oil of myrtle — rub on the involved region as often as desired.
- Oil of Bay Berry — rub liberally on the involved region three or more times daily.
- vitamin E — take 800 I.U. daily; also, apply to lesion
- beta carotene — take 25,000 I.U. daily.

- organic selenium — take 200 to 400 mcg daily.
- Juice of Oregano — drink two or more ounces twice daily.

Things to avoid
- refined vegetable oils and hydrogenated oils
- deep fried foods of all types
- sunbathing
- sun exposure at high noon

Meningitis

Meningitis is a life-threatening condition, which is defined as inflammation and infection of the brain. This is an extremely treacherous disease, which often fails to respond to even the most aggressive medical therapy. The fact is certain of the meningitis germs are entirely resistant to synthetic antibiotics. Thus, if this disorder breaks out during a crisis, the individual must be armed with other means besides drugs. What is really frightening is that outbreaks of meningitis are developing virtually everywhere. Plus, the germ which causes these epidemics is unusually aggressive. The bizarre bacteria, known as ET-15, is twice as deadly as the normal agent.

The symptoms of meningitis are fairly predictable. The major symptoms include:
- high fever
- headache
- nausea and vomiting (possibly)
- stiff neck (this is of great importance, since the flu, colds, strep throat, etc. don't present with stiff neck). Doctors know that if the individual is extremely ill, the neck should be gently moved to see if it is rigid. This distinguishes meningitis from virtually any other infection.

Note: infants don't usually develop stiff necks. The usual symptoms in infants are:
- temperature instability
- listlessness
- unusually high pitched cry (feeble cry)
- no appetite

- weak sucking response
- irritability
- vomiting and/or diarrhea

Be aware that the main issue with infants is that there is a sudden change in their normal physical condition or mental state. If their behavior is highly unusual, be suspicious of significant infection. As always, if an outbreak of meningitis occurs, see your physician immediately. The following amounts are for children over 5 years of age.

Meningitis combat kit
- oil of oregano — take a few drops under the tongue frequently, like every 15 minutes. Gently rub the neck and head with the oil of oregano (SuperStrength is preferable).
- oil of wild lavender — take 2 to 5 drops twice daily. Rub on forehead and under nose several times daily. Also, rub on the soles of the feet several times daily.
- Oregamax capsules — take as many capsules daily as possible.
- Flavin-C (as a source of immune stimulating ascorbates) — take 2 or 3 capsules as often as possible.
- bromelain (to improve blood flow to the brain) — take 2 or more capsules on an empty stomach three times daily.
- Resvitanol — take a teaspoon twice daily. In severe cases take a teaspoon at least four times daily.

Foods that help
- raw honey (easy to tolerate); consume at least three tablespoons daily
- carob molasses (well tolerated; nourishing)
- ginger root: slice and add to hot water; drink to combat nausea or upset stomach

Menstrual bleeding (heavy)
Bleeding from the vagina usually only has one cause: a bleeding uterus. It is one of the most commonly occurring conditions in women, afflicting up to 15% of the population. Chronic excessive

bleeding may lead to anemia and weakness. If unstoppable, it could result in a life-threatening crisis.

Short of a hysterectomy, medical doctors offer little successful therapy. In fact, J. Rosenfeld, M.D., writing in *American Family Physician,* January, 1996, indicates that this condition hasn't been studied thoroughly in the U. S., nor have any proven drug therapies been devised. Yet, for thousands of years primitives, as well as advanced societies, have found effective therapy among herbs. While herbs may frequently be invaluable, they don't always work. This is because the uterus may be diseased beyond repair, which leads to profuse bleeding. If bleeding is continuous or unresponsive to conservative measures, surgical intervention may be necessary.

Menstrual bleeding combat kit
• oil of fennel — take 10 drops twice daily internally.
• oil of rosemary (apply to vaginal walls)
• oil of oregano — dilute with extra virgin olive oil; apply to the vaginal walls. Also, take 2 drops twice daily under the tongue.
• oil of sage (to balance the hormone system) — take 5 to 10 drops twice daily.
• essential fatty acids (primrose or borage oils) — take 4 capsules twice daily.
• uncoated bromelain (BromaZyme) — take 2 or more capsules twice daily on an empty stomach.

Things to avoid
• refined sugar, soda pop, corn syrup, and all sweets
• caffeine, chocolate, and iced tea

Menstrual cramps
Menstrual cramps are not an inevitable consequence of being a female. There are a number of physical causes for them. Nutritional deficiency is a major factor. Nutrients which improve the function of the uterus and help prevent cramps include pantothenic acid, magnesium, vitamin E, essential fatty acids, and vitamin B_6.

Excessive cramping may also warn of uterine and/or

cervical infection. Major culprits include yeasts (Candida albicans), viruses, and bacteria, the most notorious being Chlamydia.

Menstrual cramps/difficulty combat kit
• bromelain (uncoated, i.e. BromaZyme) — take 2 or more capsules on an empty stomach twice daily.
• oil of oregano — 2 drops under the tongue twice daily.
• oil of myrtle — apply to the vaginal walls twice daily.
• oil of rosemary — apply to the vaginal walls twice daily.
Also, take 5 to 10 drops twice daily in juice or water.
• Flavin-C — take 2 or more capsules three times daily; with severe bleeding double the dosage.
• essential fatty acids (primrose or borage oils) — take 4 capsules twice daily.

Foods that help
• fatty fish (salmon, halibut, sardines, mackerel, bluefish, trout)
• unripe raw pineapple (eat the top, that is the part closest to the stem); papaya and its seeds

Things to avoid
• totally avoid chocolate, coffee, colas, and other sources of caffeine

Mercury poisoning
Mercury poisoning can occur in several ways besides touching or swallowing globs of mercury. This highly toxic metal is a component of hundreds of industrial chemicals. Billions of pounds of mercury are found in storage tanks across the United States. The fact is mercury, in the form of solid, liquid, and/or gaseous compounds, is transported via rail and truck by the megaton throughout the United States every year.

Fungicides and insecticides are often mercury based. Thus, poisoning by these chemicals may be due to mercury components.

The most commonly occurring type of mercury poisoning is due to chronic exposure. This exposure is primarily in the mouth via mercury amalgam dental fillings. Research indicates that mercury fillings poison the kidneys, brain, adrenal glands, and liver. The best means of treatment is to remove the mercury load from the body. Existing fillings should be removed and additional ones should be avoided.

All mercury compounds are aggressive poisons. They act by destroying the protein of human cells, in other words, they decimate human enzyme systems. The enzymes are absolutely critical for the existence of the body's life forces. In addition, mercury binds to cell membrane proteins, leading to the rupture of cells. Toxicity may occur via ingestion, inhalation, or direct contact with the skin. Symptoms of acute poisoning include:
• abdominal pain
• diarrhea
• nausea and vomiting
• respiratory distress
• loss of sensation
• loss of coordination
• headache

Mercury poisoning combat kit
• oil of cilantro plus coriander — take 10 drops twice daily.
• oil of cumin — take 10 drops twice daily.
• oil of rosemary — take 10 drops twice daily.
• Hercules Strength rosemary/sage/oregano herbal supplement — take 6 capsules daily.
• red grape powder — take 1 teaspoon twice daily.
• Flavin-C — take 3 capsules three times daily.
• organic selenium — take 3 capsules twice daily.
• LivaClenz — take 10 drops twice daily.

Migraines (see Headaches)

Mite allergy
Dust mite allergy is a primary cause of respiratory distress, sinus problems, asthma, and other common disorders. It is not the only cause of this illness, but it contributes to it in a major way. As described by T. Johnson, M. D., in *American Family Physician*, fully 1 in 10 individuals and 9 of 10 asthmatics react to these pests.

The problem of mites has been aggravated by modern living: they love living along with humans. They love our homes and thrive at the temperature in which we thrive. In particular, they flourish in the moist tropics and in subtropical regions, like the southeastern United States.

One rather shocking fact is that mites don't just reside on the ground or in dust. They seek to reside as close to the human body as possible. This is why they flourish in bedding, where they have a captive source of nourishment for several hours. A pillow alone may house as many as a quarter of a million of these pests. A study published in 1995 by Australian researchers discovered that mites thrive in our clothes. The researchers found that there are enough mites and mite secretions on virtually anyone to provoke allergic reactions or respiratory problems in susceptible individuals. Perhaps even more grotesque is the fact that other research documents how mites thrive on our bodies, that is on the skin and in the hair, despite normal hygiene. Therefore, additional tactics must be utilized to destroy these vermin.

Essential oils kill mites effectively. Top anti-mite essential oils include the oils of wild oregano, lavender, bay leaf, and rosemary. The most aggressive of these is oil of oregano. Add a combination of these oils to body shampoos or pump soap for washing to help keep mites off the body.

Mite combat kit
• oil of oregano — take 2 drops under the tongue whenever needed; add to diffuser and volatilize into air.
• Might at Night™ (a special formula of potent essential oils) — rub anywhere on the body as needed. Note: mites may live on the skin, hair, and scalp.
• oil of bay leaf — take 5 drops daily and add to diffuser; pump spray into air and add to wash cycle.
• oil of rosemary — diffuse into air; add to wash cycle.

Other ideas
• wash all clothes and bedding in hot water. Only hot water washes kill mites, as they can survive cold/warm washes. Add bleach when appropriate. Add also oil of oregano, a few drops per wash cycle.
• rub oil of oregano, oil of bay leaf, and/or oil of lavender on the

skin before dressing. This will allow the oils to "fumigate" the clothes throughout the day. This is particularly valuable for wool clothes, which can't be washed in hot water. Wool clothes retain the greatest numbers of mites.

Mold allergy/poisoning

This section is perhaps the most important of any in this book. Mold poisoning is a monumental cause of illness, disability, disease, and death. It is rarely diagnosed, in fact, it is almost never considered. Yet, it is pervasive and insidious and frequently causes human distress, perhaps for years or even decades before it is recognized if ever.

Did you know that it is virtually certain that molds are the most dangerous of all germs and that they have caused throughout history a greater degree of disability and death than the Plague? It was M. K. Matossian, in her book, *Poisons of the Past: Molds, Epidemics, and History*, who wrote that molds are wreaking havoc on the human race, causing sudden death, physical exhaustion, and mental aberrations. Regarding the latter, she mentions how mold poisons, through contamination of stored food, caused massive outbreaks of psychosis, often affecting entire cities. Matossian further writes that it was ergotism, a form of mold poisoning, which caused the illnesses that led to the notorious Salem Witch Trials. These poisons are capable of completely disabling the neurological systems, as well as the immune system, making the individual extremely ill.

Case history: A 28 year-old woman was admitted to the psychiatric ward for acute psychosis, which developed after she went on a sugar and chocolate binge. Doctors noticed she also had a rash on her feet, legs, and hands, which appeared to be a fungal infection. Her mother insisted that the doctors consider using an antifungal approach to help her daughter. All sugar and starch were eliminated from her diet. Oil of oregano, a natural antifungal agent, was administered aggressively; 20 drops three times daily. She was also given Royal Kick, 4 capsules three times daily, to rebuild her adrenal glands. Within 48 hours the patient's behavior improved to such an extent that she was released. In addition, the rash had improved significantly. Thus, a medical and social disaster was averted.

Mold contaminated foods are not the only culprits. The molds found in the air and, particularly, inside homes and other buildings may be highly toxic. What's more, they can readily invade the body, infecting virtually any region or organ. Apparently, the toxic effects of these "household molds" is particularly dangerous for children. The CDC recently reported a high number of illnesses, as well as deaths, due to an indoor mold known as *Stachybotrus atra*. This mold produces potent chemicals, which cause immune depression and internal bleeding. Children have been killed by inhaling these mold poisons. They bleed to death into their lungs. However, untold thousands more have been poisoned, many fatally, and, again, no one suspects it. The dilemma is so serious that the American Academy of Pediatrics issued a warning to all doctors entitled, "Toxic Effects of Indoor Mold." It doesn't take much to induce damage. Just a tiny quantity, less than the amount placed on a pinhead, is enough to decimate an individual. J. S. Marr, M. D., writing in the *JAMA*, notes that these "extremely potent...poisons...cause numerous diseases in trifling amounts." He further describes that the Tenth Plague of ancient Egypt was probably due to such mold toxins, which proliferated as a result of floods. The fact is the current outbreaks in the United States are largely due to the plethora of severe floods, which have decimated numerous regions such as South Texas, Central Iowa, North Dakota, Missouri, Ohio, and parts of California. Symptoms of mold poisoning are highly variable. However, the most common manifestations include:

- unquenchable thirst
- poor appetite (or excessive appetite for sugar)
- bizarre heat sensations (hot flashes)
- cold extremities, worsened when eating certain foods
- intolerance to weather extremes, hot or cold
- tingling sensations
- joint pain and/or spinal stiffness
- itching or redness of the skin

- swelling and/or blistering of the skin
- hysterical and/or psychotic behavior
- loss of hearing
- headaches and/or sinus pain
- nosebleeds
- exhaustion
- asthma-like symptoms
- skin eruptions, eczema, and/or psoriasis
- nausea and/or vomiting
- dark colored smelly stools
- depression
- internal bleeding
- apathy
- inability to cope

Not all of these symptoms need to necessarily be present for infestation to be proven. If you have 6 or more of these symptoms, mold toxicity is highly likely. A score of 10 or more indicates massive mold contamination.

Mold allergy/poisoning combat kit

- oil of oregano — take 2 or 3 drops under the tongue twice daily plus an additional 10 drops twice daily in juice or water. For more severe exposure take more often.
- wild oregano herb (Oregamax capsules) — take 3 capsules twice daily.
- oil of cumin — take 5 to 10 drops twice daily.
- Lactobacillus — take several capsules daily. Take at a different time from taking oregano oil.
- oil of bay leaf — take 5 drops twice daily.
- organic selenium, zinc, and manganese — to activate the mold detoxification systems.
- Flavin-C — crude ascorbic acid plus bioflavonoids to activate white blood cells, 2 or 3 capsules twice daily.
- Fungi-Clenz (special formula of natural spice/herb oils for removing fungal residues and toxins from the body) — take 5 or more drops twice daily in juice or water (or under the tongue).

Note: the oils should be volatilized to cleanse the air and penetrate the lungs directly. Use a diffuser or atomizer.

Foods that help
* garlic and onions (raw)
* cloves and cinnamon

Things to avoid
* rye of all types
* wheat and corn

Mononucleosis

Mononucleosis, known commonly as mono, is caused by a virus belonging to the herpes family. The virus usually attacks adolescents and college students and is readily transmitted sexually, primarily through kissing.

The mono virus specifically attacks the lymphatic system. This is why swollen lymph glands is a major sign of this illness. The liver and spleen are a part of the lymph system and are also aggressively attacked. Antibiotics are of no use in this condition and usually aggravate it.

Mono combat kit
* oil of oregano — take 2 or more drops under the tongue several times daily. Rub on feet, buttocks, and abdomen.
* Oregamax capsules — take 3 capsules three times daily.
* oil of cilantro/coriander — take 10 drops twice daily in juice or water.
* oil of cumin — take 10 or more drops daily.

Things to avoid
* alcoholic beverages
* antibiotics
* prescription pain killers, aspirin, and acetaminophen

Mosquito bites

Mosquitoes, seemingly mere pests in North America, are the number one direct transmitter of infectious disease globally. They cause a wide gamut of diseases, including yellow fever, dengue fever, malaria, worm infections, and encephalitis.

There is a simple way to prevent these infections: avoid getting bitten. This implies the use of repellents. However, the commercial repellents are themselves poisonous. According to Dr. S. Fradin, author of "Mosquitoes and Mosquito Repellents: a Clinician's Guide", published in the *Annals of Internal Medicine*, 1998, there is a repellent that is equally as effective as the synthetics. Called *Bite Blocker*, it is apparently 97% effective.

Another therapy is to detoxify the bite as soon as it occurs. This is accomplished through the application of essential oils. The oils of oregano, cumin, lavender, bay leaf, and bay berry all offer anti-toxic actions.

Mosquito combat kit
- oil of oregano — apply to bite region and take a drop or two under the tongue.
- raw garlic — crush cloves and apply small amount to bite.
- mosquito netting
- oil of wild lavender — as a healing agent, apply to any bite.

Things to avoid
- perfumes

Muscle soreness and weakness
This can happen to anyone. Usually, it is a symptom of over-exertion or infectious disease. Certain illnesses, such as chronic fatigue and fibromyalgia, may be manifested by it. Common causes are chronic stress, infection, allergic reactions, and nutritional deficiency. Poor circulation and blood pooling add to this aggravation.

Muscle soreness/weakness combat kit
- bromelain (BromaZyme) — take 3 or more capsules twice daily on an empty stomach.
- sea salt — consume a heaping teaspoonful daily in food.
- oil of oregano — take 10 drops twice daily in juice or water.
- oil of rosemary — take 10 drops twice daily in juice or water.
- oil of sage — rub on sore muscles and on soles of feet.
- chromium, chelated (or from Resvitanol) — take 3 capsules twice daily.

Foods that help
- papaya plus the seeds
- salted roasted nuts, especially almonds and filberts

Nail bed infection

Known medically as *paronychia*, this infection is usually caused by a fungus, notably Candida albicans. Less commonly, bacteria are the culprits. In either case it is a painful infection, which may persist unless it is aggressively treated. It is manifested by swelling around the nail bed, redness, and extreme pain.

Nail bed infection combat kit
- oil of oregano — take 3 drops under the tongue three times daily. Soak the finger in a solution of oil of oregano and olive oil. Or, simply rub the oil twice daily on the involved region.
- oil of lavender — rub on the involved region.
- bromelain — take 3 or 4 capsules three times daily on an empty stomach.
- Flavin-C — take 3 capsules twice daily.

Things to avoid
- nail polish and artificial nails
- harsh soaps
- sugar and other sweets

Nasal polyps

The primary cause of nasal polyps appears to be a vitamin deficiency, that is a lack of vitamin A. Zinc deficiency may also play a role. Food allergies are an aggravating factor. However, infection, that is chronic infection, is a more likely cause. This makes sense, since both vitamin A and zinc are required for normal immune function.

Nasal polyp combat kit
- vitamin A — 25,000 to 50,000 I.U. daily for two months; then, 10,000 to 25,000 I.U. per day.

- zinc — 50 mg daily.
- BromaZyme — take 3 capsules on an empty stomach twice daily.
- oil of oregano — 2 or 4 drops under the tongue twice daily.
- Black seed-plus — take 2 or more capsules twice daily. Also, open capsules and add contents to food or chew on the seeds.

Nausea

This is one of the most uncomfortable of all conditions. It is caused by inflammation in the gut, although head injuries also lead to nausea. The inflammation may be due to infection, stress, chemical poisoning, alcohol toxicity, drug reactions, pesticide/herbicide intoxication, or allergic reactions. Nausea of pregnancy is another consideration. In fact, nausea is one of the earliest symptoms of pregnancy. It is also the primary symptom of motion sickness.

Nausea also has an ominous component; it may be a sign of intestinal or stomach cancer. Whatever the cause, herbs and spices are effective remedies. Even in cancer, they often relieve the agony.

Nausea combat kit
- ginger root, either fresh, dehydrated, or capsules: take as needed.
- oil of ginger (from the entire ginger plant emulsified in extra virgin olive oil) — take 2 or 3 drops with each meal or as needed.
- HerbSorb capsules — take one or two capsules as needed until nausea abates.
- oil of fennel — take 5 drops in warm water once or twice daily.
- Essence of Orange Blossom — delicate and soothing; add two tablespoons to hot water and drink as a tea.
- Juice of Oregano — drink an ounce as often as needed.
- Black seed-plus — take 2 capsules two or more times daily.
- pressure point wrist bands

Things to avoid
- Food: rest the gut as long as possible or until the nausea abates.
- alcohol of any type
- synthetic chemicals, aspirin, and radiation

Nerve gas poisoning

This seems unlikely, yet it happened in Japan. When sarin gas was released in the subway system, thousands of individuals were overcome; some permanently. Nerve gas poisonings could just as easily occur here, whether deliberate or accidental. As reported in the *Chicago Tribune* in December, 1998, some 150 gallons of the deadly nerve gas sarin, the same one that poisoned the Japanese, spilled at an Army incineration facility in Utah. Apparently, no one was hurt and the spill was contained or at least so Army officials claim. Yet, if this would have become airborne, it was enough gas to destroy all of Salt Lake City, a mere 20 miles away.

While nerve gas poisoning is unlikely, if it does occur, no one will be prepared; the government offers no curative aid. However, major incidents affecting thousands of individuals will assuredly occur, both in the Western world and developing countries. Thus, the following protocol provides the individual with the best odds for survival.

Nerve gas combat kit
- gas mask and protective clothing
- oil of cumin — take 10 drops every few minutes.
- oil of rosemary — 10 drops every few minutes; take also under the tongue 2 drops frequently.
- oil of oregano — take 2 drops under the tongue every few minutes.
- organic selenium — take 200 mcg every two hours for two or three days, then take 600 to 800 mcg daily. Only organically bound selenium can be consumed in these quantities; be sure of your source, because synthetic selenium is toxic.

LivaClenz (to protect the liver from toxic chemical damage) — take 10 to 20 drops twice daily.

Juice of Oregano (to maintain physical strength and prevent collapse) — drink several ounces daily.

oil of rosemary (prevents brain damage) — 20 or more drops daily.

NukeProtect — take 2 capsules several times daily.

Nervousness/Irritability

Virtually everyone has experienced a bout of nervousness. Yet, it becomes a disease when it is a daily event.

Certain individuals seem to never relax. This may not be exclusively a mental issue, as it is a sign of a damaged coping mechanism. This coping mechanism is controlled by a set of glands known as the adrenal glands. Thus, persistent nervousness is nearly always a sign of adrenal insufficiency. Symptoms of emotional instability, which includes frustration, anger, crying spells, anxiety, panic attacks, depression, and extreme sensitivity, are all indicative of weak adrenals. For further information see the tests/symptom analysis in Dr. Ingram's *Self-Test Nutrition Guide* or check the self-testing web site, **NutritionTest.com.**

Nervousness/irritability combat kit
• St. John's wort (wild and unprocessed) — take 2 to 4 capsules in the a.m.
• oil of lavender (wild type in extra virgin olive oil) — 2 drops under the tongue twice daily. Also, rub on the chest, neck, and soles of feet.
• Royal Kick premium grade royal jelly — take 4 to 6 capsules every morning. Use more if needed to combat stress or anxiety.
• oil or juice of sage — add a few drops to fruit juice or hot water as a tea. If using sage juice, add a tablespoon to juice or hot water.

Foods that help
• salty healthy snacks like salted roasted nuts or salted fresh meat

Nosebleeds
Nosebleeds occur most commonly in children and teenagers. The major cause is nutritional deficiency, although infection and trauma are also involved. Nosebleeds warn of deficiencies of calcium, copper, vitamin C, zinc, folic acid, vitamin K, and bioflavonoids. Infections that may cause it include those induced by molds, yeasts, bacteria, parasites, and viruses. Mold intolerance is particularly likely to cause nose bleeds, because mold toxins, due to their poisonous actions on the liver, are a major cause of internal bleeding.

Nosebleed combat kit
- oil of oregano — drip it into the nose. Take 2 drops under the tongue every 15 minutes until bleeding halts. Also, take a few drops under the tongue as an anti-mold therapy on a daily basis.
- chelated calcium — take 500 mg every 15 minutes for at least 2 hours, then 2000 mg per day for one week. Then, take 1000 mg daily as a maintenance. For best results take calcium in divided dosages, including a dose of at least 500 mg at bedtime.
- Flavin-C — take 6 or more capsules daily. Also, open a capsule and place contents in mouth or under tongue; repeat as needed.
- red grape powder (Resvitanol) — take 6 or more capsules daily.
- Lactobacillus (to antagonize the molds) — take as directed.
- Oregamax capsules (mold antagonist and natural calcium/magnesium supplement) — take 3 capsules twice daily.

Nuclear catastrophe (see also Radiation poisoning)
This is virtually impossible to prepare for. However, by utilizing the information in this section you will have among the best tools available for survival.
There is a high likelihood of a nuclear catastrophe in the United States. This is because of the risks of nuclear power plant accidents, not from some outside military threat. The United States has the largest number of nuclear power plants in the world, over 100, and dozens of these reactors are at a high risk for leaks and/or accidents. Other risks include accidents during the transport of nuclear wastes. Currently, all nuclear power plants leak radiation, negatively affecting at a minimum anyone living within a 20 mile radius of the plant. A study in England found a 10-fold increased occurrence of leukemia in plant workers, plus there is a higher than normal risk for individuals living in close proximity. Marketed as "clean fuel", it is far from clean, since nuclear releases permanently damage the human body as well as any portion of the earth contacted. Do not be fooled by marketing language. Nuclear power plants continuously release into the environment poisonous gases as well as water. Plus, unless aging and friable plants are systematically and permanently closed, a nuclear release/accident of massive proportions is a virtual certainty in this country.

Computer mishaps merely heighten the risks. In March, 1999, the Russian government asked the U. S. government to provide some 20 million dollars in funds to ready their nuclear plants for potential 21st century disasters. Yet, in the USA life-threatening contamination already exists. For instance, the *U.S News & World Report*, August 30, 1999, documents the existence of radioactive parking lots and streets in Paducah, Kentucky, a contamination resulting from plutonium-containing trucks parked there.

The major way to become poisoned by nuclear ions is through the respiratory passages or the ingestion of water and food. Remember, these ions are primarily minerals, that is they are large ions (bigger molecularly than vitamins), so passage through the skin is less of a problem than inhalation and/or ingestion. Thus, one of the keys to survival is to block and/or prevent inhalation and ingestion. However, radioactive ions may exert direct toxicity to the surface of the body, causing massive skin damage, ulcerations, and radiation burns.

Radiation harms the body by destroying cells, particularly the highly friable cells of the immune system. Nutritional therapy helps protect the cells through every means possible, and antioxidant nutrients are the number one tool available.

Nuclear catastrophe survival/combat kit
• oil of cumin — take 20 or more drops (one dropper full) every few minutes.
• oil of rosemary — take 20 or more drops every few minutes both internally and under the tongue.
• Juice of Oregano, Juice of Sage, Juice of Rosemary — very important; drink up to a bottle of each daily. Highly protective against radiation poisoning, Juice of Oregano was used successfully to save the lives of Chernobyl victims.
• oil of oregano — take 10 or more drops every few minutes plus several drops under the tongue every few minutes.
• resveratrol-rich red grape powder (Resvitanol) — highly valuable for total body protection; take as much as possible. For highest intake consume the bulk type; take a teaspoon every hour initially, then a few teaspoons daily. For quickest absorption hold the Resvitanol in the mouth for a few moments before swallowing.

With capsules take 4 to 6 capsules every hour.
• organic selenium — take 200 mcg every hour. Do this only for one week, then take 600 mcg daily.
• vitamin E (as mixed tocopherols and/or tocotrienols) — take 400 I.U. every hour for one to two days; then 2400 I.U. daily.
• Black seed-plus —take 3 or more capsules every few hours.
• Oil of Bay Berry (for radiation burns) — apply liberally to the injured region.
• raw honey (for radiation burns) — apply as needed
• Aloe vera gel — use topically on radiation burns/wounds.
• portable gas mask with anti-nuclear ion cartridges
• water filtration straws

Note: with the above mentioned supplements the more that is taken the greater is the protection. Be excessive; consume large amounts of these items in the event of a nuclear catastrophe. A simple way to get the minimum degree of protection is via special anti-nuclear supplements. These supplements were created just as this book is going to press. Called NukeProtect™, these supplements provide the minimal necessary protection:
• NukeProtect essential oil formula (special blend of oregano, rosemary, ginger, cumin, and sage oils) — take 10 or more drops three times daily. Also, use NukeProtect juice formula.
• NukeProtect super-protective capsules (iodine/selenium formula) — in the event of major exposure take 2 or more capsules every hour. For continued protection take 6 or more capsules daily.

Foods that help
• anything rich in saturated fat like whole milk, butter, beef, avocados, nut butters, etc. These heavy fats block the toxicity of radioactive ions, whereas vegetable oils accelerate them.
• fatty fish
• Brazil nuts (because of their rich supply of selenium)
• papaya and kiwi fruit
• tomato paste (lycopene, the tomato pigment, intercepts nuclear ions; be sure to add olive oil to the paste, as lycopene absorption is dependent upon dietary fats)

Things to avoid
• refined vegetable oils of any type
• iron of any type (except that naturally occurring in food)
• all contaminated foods, especially meat products and milk (animals concentrate radioactivity from contaminated soil/grass)

Pesticide/herbicide poisoning

It is estimated that a minimum of 500,000 individuals develop severe pesticide poisoning every year. This is a conservative estimate; the number is probably far higher: in the tens of millions.

Pesticides are ubiquitous, although they were unknown on this planet 100 years ago. They contaminate virtually every square inch of the earth. According to M. J. Bayer, medical toxicologist at the Connecticut Poison Control Center, these chemicals are "routinely sprayed over fields and farms", poisoning thousands of individuals, especially rural workers.

A mysterious flu has been afflicting farmers for decades. Previously attributed to molds or other germs housed in grain elevators, now the cause has been elucidated: toxic farm chemicals. Researchers publishing in *The Practitioner* (March, 1993) found that when 34 people with known pesticide poisoning were analyzed, all had flu like symptoms. These symptoms included debilitating fatigue, muscle and joint aches, and severe depression. While the farmers' ailments were usually misdiagnosed as the flu, arthritis, or psychological disorders, the cause was exclusively pesticide poisoning, either chronic or acute.

Repeated exposure to pesticides is life threatening, because these chemicals poison the brain and nervous system, disrupting their impulses to vital internal organs such as the heart, lungs, and kidneys. Yet, even a single exposure can kill. What happens is the pesticide poisons enzymes in the nervous system, which are responsible for breaking down neurotransmitters. Without these enzymes, the neurotransmitters accumulate within the brain and nerves to toxic levels, causing them to go haywire. This should be no surprise, since this poisoning of the nervous system is how these chemicals kill pests. Symptoms of sudden massive exposure include:
• massive sweating

- very slow heart rate
- twitching, often violent
- vomiting and nausea
- abdominal contractions
- convulsions and/or seizures
- severe respiratory distress

Daily exposure to pesticides is a more realistic problem than exposure from a sudden disaster, like an overturned tanker car or a chemical plant release. As is reported by *Mother Jones* magazine, July/August, 1998, unwittingly, virtually all individuals are being exposed and we don't realize it, at least this is true for those who fly. Tens of millions of individuals experience vague sensations, cold sweats, claustrophobia, head pain, ear ache, sinus trouble, nausea, or flu symptoms, during or shortly after a flight. However, few realize that these symptoms are often due to pesticide poisoning rather than from germs. In all likelihood the plane you board was treated with pesticide spray recently, perhaps the day that you enter it. Numerous airlines confirmed to the magazine that they regularly or occasionally spray their planes with pesticides, and this includes some of the world's most prominent airlines: American, Continental, Delta, TWA, US Airways, United Airlines, and Northwest. What's more, these are domestic flights, not international. When questioned about the reason for spraying airplanes and passengers with toxic compounds, the explanation is "to kill mice."

Certainly, some of this pesticide is absorbed into the traveler's body, either via inhalation or through the skin. The skin is like a sponge, and it is unable to protect us. Becky Riley from the Northwest Coalition of Alternatives to Pesticides describes this dangerous practice thusly, "Pesticides break down slowly in the enclosed, poorly ventilated aircraft...passengers are *sealed in a chamber that has been gassed and sit there for hours* (italics mine)." According to Dr. Jack Thrasher, immunotoxicologist of Alto, New Mexico, the so-called preventive spraying of pesticides on airliners amounts to the "practice of insanity." He notes that one of the typical airline pesticides, Tralomethrin, can cause severe allergic reactions, even asthma attacks. Thrasher further proclaims that the airlines "have no business spraying pesticide" on their planes and that the practice isn't even required by law. What's more, federal agencies, such as the Department of Transportation, are on record stating that they not only fail to require spraying but have no idea why the airlines do so. However, their "sterile" attitude to this crisis is edified by Bill Mosley, public affairs specialist at the DOT, who says "there is no prohibition against (the airlines) doing as they wish." Yet, it was Dr. Donald Hopkins, former Assistant Surgeon General, who stated categorically that the practice of spraying noxious pesticides on planes was not only useless but also highly dangerous. Furthermore, he noted, it has never been proven to effectively control pest growth or prevent disease. Yet, fatalities have likely occurred on airlines due to pesticide reactions and have been "misdiagnosed" as heart attacks. Pesticides are the most poisonous chemicals known. For instance, until 1996 Northwest Airlines used a compound known as *Bolt*, which outright poisons the nervous system: one of the consequences of such a poisoning is sudden death/heart attack. What's more, a report by the *Journal of Pesticide Reform* describes the well known birth defect-inducing action of this chemical. The pesticides currently used are far from safe and have been implicated in causing birth defects, cancer, and reduced sperm counts as well as neurological disorders. Dave Noetzel, an entomologist at the University of Minnesota, also finds the practice of poisoning the interior of airliners with pesticides abhorrent, stating that at best "it is overkill" and that, in fact, it is a "meaningless procedure." In other words, the public is put at extreme risk without cause. It was Bill Plapp who also noted that this practice should be deemed illegal, because "people should have the right to transportation without being subjected to a health hazard."

A United Airlines pilot recently reported that many of the airline's employees are against the pesticide contamination. Yet, their concerns have apparently been ignored, since this silent poisoning continues.

Pesticides are highly toxic to brain tissue, and they tend to concentrate there. An article published in *Neurology*, May, 1998, describes how farm chemicals dramatically increase the risk of neurological disease. The researchers found that farmers who regularly use pesticides are over four times more likely to develop

Parkinson's disease than controls. This clearly illustrates the extreme toxicity of pesticides to the human organism.

Remember that pesticides are fulminant nervous system poisons. Many of them are molecularly the same as the nerve gases synthesized during the World War II. Do not use them carelessly. In fact, do not use them at all.

The symptoms produced by pesticides/herbicides depend upon the type of chemical. However, the primary symptoms include:

• spasticity of the lungs, increased bronchial secretions, suffocation on secretions, swelling in the lungs.
• radical drop in heart rate or radical rise in heart rate
• nausea, vomiting, diarrhea
• excessive sweating; cold, clammy feeling
• excessive tearing
• inability to hold urine (incontinence)
• muscle twitching/jerking, weakness, and paralysis
• headache, confusion, convulsions, and coma

Note: beware if you suddenly become sick for no apparent reason. Pesticides fail to degrade quickly and residues may remain throughout the plane even without obvious spraying. Plus, the planes are sprayed repeatedly.

Pesticide detoxification/combat kit
• oil of cumin — take 10 or more drops several times daily.
• oil of fennel — take 10 or more drops twice daily.
• oil of oregano — take 2 drops under the tongue often, like 5 or more times daily. Also, take 10 drops twice daily in juice or water.
• Juice of Oregano — drink as much as possible, like a bottle or half bottle daily.
• red grape powder (Resvitanol) — take 4 to 6 capsules three times daily or a teaspoon of the bulk powder three times daily.
• organic selenium — take 100 or 200 mcg every few hours until the poisoning is resolved. Then, take 200 to 400 mcg daily. Do not use sodium selenite or selenious acid, which may be toxic.
• chlorella — consume as much as possible.
• vinegar — drink 6 or more ounces daily added to juice or water.
• Nutri-Sense drink mix (to provide nerve regenerating natural B

vitamins and phospholipids) — take 3 heaping tablespoons twice daily.
• LivaClenz — take 10 drops twice daily. After a week or two reduce the amount to 5 drops twice daily (note: if you take this, you don't need to take the oils of fennel or cumin).

Foods that help
• pure extra virgin olive oil (binds the chemicals and aids in their elimination through the liver) — drink a cup per day for a few days.

Pinworms

This is one of the most common causes of intestinal pain and other gut symptoms in children. As many as 30% of children globally suffer from this condition. The infection occurs almost exclusively in children under 14. Early symptoms are abdominal pain, constipation, and itching of the anus. Severe itching of the anus is common, and, when children scratch this region, feces and pinworm eggs become trapped under the nails. Thus, when the child eats, he/she becomes reinfected and spreads the infection to others. The fingernails house the eggs, and if they are not kept trimmed, the child may transmit the infection to virtually anyone, including family members, friends, and other school children.

Pinworm combat kit
• oil of oregano — take 3 to 5 drops twice daily in juice or water.
• oil of cumin — take 5 to 10 drops twice daily (it is disguised best in tomato juice). Also, rub on the anus; wash hands thoroughly.
• oil of bay leaf — rub on anus and buttocks.
• oil of rosemary — rub on anus and buttocks.
• HerbSorb — take 2 or more capsules twice daily.
• oil of fennel — take 10 drops daily.
Note: in the event of infection bedding must be thoroughly washed. Soap alone is not sufficient to guarantee sterility. When washing bedding or underwear, add a sterilizing agent, such as chlorine or, preferably, antiseptic essential oils such as oil of oregano, oil of bay leaf, oil of cinnamon, or oil of clove.

Plague

Odds are low for a Plague outbreak in the United States. However, this dangerous illness is increasing in frequency, especially in the southwestern states. Serious outbreaks have occurred recently in India, Africa, and China.

Plague is caused by a bacteria, which is transmitted to humans via the bites of fleas. The fleas usually contract the germ from rodents. However, squirrels are the major reservoir in the western United States.

In some respects the Plague is one of the easiest diseases to prevent. This is because with natural antiseptics any potential bite or lesion can be effectively treated immediately. By sterilizing any suspect lesion, the development of Plague may be aborted.

Plague combat kit
• oil of oregano (SuperStrength may be necessary) — apply to any suspect lesion. Also, take 2 or more drops under the tongue several times daily. If needed, take 5 to 10 drops in juice or water twice daily.
• Oregamax capsules — take 4 capsules three times daily.
• Flavin-C — take 2 capsules three times daily.
• Black seed-plus — take 3 or more capsules three times daily.
• Oil of Bay Berry — rub on any open wound or lesion.
• BromaZyme — take 3 capsules three times daily on an empty stomach.

Foods that help
• raw garlic/onion
• crude raw honey

Pneumonia

This is a potentially fatal condition, which usually afflicts the elderly. However, increasingly it is afflicting individuals of all ages. Currently, an outbreak of pneumonia is undermining the health of middle aged individuals as well as children. The problem is that certain individuals, many in the prime of their lives, suffer either health devastation and/or death as a result of what should be a temporary or curable illness. Pneumonia doesn't have to kill.

Case History: Mrs. M., mother of my associate, was placed in a nursing home, basically to die. The 80 year-old but spry lady had just been transferred from a hospital and was in a weakened state. Complaining of a relentless cough, shortness of breath, and lack of appetite, it was obvious that she had contracted a communal germ in the nursing home and was quickly developing pneumonia; nurses discovered that her lungs were filled with fluid. It appeared she was going to die. Her daughter, with my blessings, added two drops of oil of oregano to a glass of water. Handing it to her coughing and feverish, mother she said, "Take this, doctor's orders." Grudgingly, she swallowed the concoction. By the evening the fever broke, she began eating vigorously, and slept without discomfort. By the next day the pneumonia symptoms had completely disappeared.

Pneumonia combat kit

- oil of oregano — take 2 or more drops several times daily. Also, take 5 or more drops twice daily.
- oil of myrtle — rub oil on chest, face, and soles of feet. Take 5 drops twice daily in juice or water.
- oil of lavender — rub on face, chest, soles of feet, and/or spine.
- Flavin-C — 3 capsules three times daily (or more often, if necessary)
- Oregamax capsules — 3 capsules three or more times daily.
- oil of rosemary — add to a diffuser or atomizer; also, take 5 to 10 drops twice daily.
- Black seed-plus — take 2 capsules several times daily.

Poison ivy, oak, and sumac

This condition is virtually impossible to cure with medical therapy. There simply is no effective drug for it.

This is not the case with natural remedies. A number of agents halt the itching as well as reverse the toxicity of these poisonous plants. Reliable remedies include oil of oregano, oil of lavender, tea tree oil, camomile extracts, and aloe vera. However, oil of oregano has the supremacy. It halts itching on contact, plus it dissolves the poisonous resins, which are notoriously difficult to dislodge. This is largely due to the fact that the oil is an effective natural solvent, and, thus, it dissolutes the noxious resins, neutralizing them as well as allowing their removal through washing them from the body.

Be aware that direct contact with the skin is not the only way to contract these conditions. According to *Hippocrates Magazine*, July, 1998, the resins from these plants stick to footwear, clothing, and even the fur of animals. Thus, it is advisable to wash thoroughly all contaminated objects. Add oil of oregano to the wash cycle. It will help dissolve or neutralize the resin.

If oil of oregano and/or tea tree oil are unavailable, a few over-the-counter remedies might help. Calamine lotion and Aveeno oatmeal cream or powder are the best. Don't use cortisone creams. According to Dr. D. Harris, a Stanford University dermatologist, they are "worthless."

Poison plant resin combat kit
• oil of oregano — apply topically as often as needed. Take 2 drops twice daily sublingually.
• oil of lavender — apply topically once or twice daily.
• tea tree oil — apply topically only.
• camomile or aloe vera cream — apply as needed.

Foods that help
• Make a chicken or beef broth heavy in garlic and onions. Chop several onions and a head or two of garlic cloves into the soup and boil until well dissolved. Drink several cups daily.

Poor appetite
Poor appetite could be caused by stress. Yet, ironically, stress in certain individuals leads to a ravenous appetite. Nutritional deficiency is another major cause. Deficiencies of certain key nutrients impair the flow of digestive juices, and this reduces the desire for wholesome food. For reasons yet to be determined the individual may have a poor appetite for healthy food, while craving instead poor quality food such as chips, pop, luncheon meats, etc.

Poor appetite is a cardinal sign of vitamin deficiency. A lack of thiamine halts stomach acid production and impairs the body's ability to process sugar. Niacin deficiency virtually aborts the body's ability to produce energy, so sorely needed for proper digestion. A lack of vitamin B_6 greatly impairs the digestion and processing of protein. Vitamin D deficiency leads to a malabsorption of fat and greatly impedes calcium absorption. Thus, poor appetite represents a vicious cycle; the individual is already deficient and by failing to eat properly, he/she becomes severely deficient. The result will certainly be impaired health and, in the extreme, anorexia, which can be fatal.

Appetite stimulation kit
• HerbSorb eastern spice formula (to stimulate the flow of digestive juices) — take 2 capsules with each meal.
• Nutri-Sense natural B vitamin drink mix — take 3 tablespoons once or twice daily in juice or water.
• premium grade royal jelly (Royal Kick) — take 4 capsules in the morning.
• red grape powder (Resvitanol) — take 2 or 3 capsules with every meal.
• Oregamax capsules — take 2 or 3 capsules with every meal.

Poor breast milk
Regardless of the circumstances breast feeding women have a handy tool, that is if the milk is delivered in abundance. Milk flow can be stimulated, merely by eating certain foods and taking safe/edible herbs and/or spices. In particular, the spices appear to be the most effective for inducing milk production. Apparently, they operate by activating body metabolism.

Breast milk stimulation kit
• oil of fennel — take 5 to 10 drops twice daily or more often if needed.
• oil of cilantro/coriander — take 5 to 10 drops twice daily.
• Resvitanol — take one or more teaspoons twice daily.

• Nutri-Sense — take 3 heaping tablespoons once or, preferably, twice daily in milk or juice.
• Black seed-plus — take 3 or more capsules twice daily.
• primrose oil — take 5 or more capsules twice daily.

Foods that help
• avocados — at least 2 per day
• steak — eat the largest portion available
• fennel seed tea with raw honey
• raw honey and/or carob molasses — take two tablespoons daily; They are mild laxatives, so eat to tolerance.
• tangy or aromatic spices, notably fennel seed, anise seed, rosemary, black seed, and coriander seed
• pumpkin/squash seeds
• fatty fish such as salmon, halibut, and trout (must be from relatively unpolluted waters)

Postnasal drip (see Sinus attacks)

Prostatitis
This is defined as inflammation of the prostate. The inflammation may result from infection, toxicity, and/or nutritional imbalances. Nutrient deficiencies of greatest importance include a lack of vitamin D, selenium, vitamin A, vitamin C, and zinc. Prostatitis can also be caused by a host of germs. Toxicity is another cause, that is the poisoning of the tissues by various noxious chemicals. Solvents are particularly likely to poison the prostate. All of these factors lead to inflammation and swelling.

Heavy metal poisoning is another cause of prostate disorders. In particular, cadmium damages the prostate. In fact, both prostatitis and prostate cancer may be directly related to the ill effects of this metal. This is because cadmium blocks the absorption and utilization of zinc, a mineral essential for the function of this gland. Normal enzyme function in the prostate is zinc dependent, and cadmium disrupts the ability of zinc to attach to the enzymes. Taking supplemental zinc may aid in displacing cadmium from the enzymes, helping return their function to normal.

Prostatitis combat kit
- Oil of Bay Berry — take 5 drops twice daily in juice or water.
- saw palmetto berry — take as directed.
- oil of fennel — take 10 to 20 drops twice daily in juice or water.
- oil of oregano — take 2 or more drops under the tongue daily.
- cranberry extract or Resvitanol (resveratrol-rich red grape concentrate) – take as needed.
- zinc chelate — 75 mg daily.

Foods that help
- pumpkin/squash seeds (raw is preferable)
- sardines, salmon, herring (for the fatty acid/vitamin D content)

Puncture wounds

This is one of the most treacherous of all illnesses, largely because the wound is difficult to access. In other words, it is difficult to completely cleanse the wound(s) of germs that may cause serious infection.

Puncture wounds are notoriously associated with a condition commonly known as "lock jaw", for which we now receive tetanus shots. The word tetanus derives from the name of the bacteria which causes lock jaw, *Clostridium tetani*. While the tetanus shot has virtually eliminated this disorder, it is of little value in a crisis. This is because puncture wounds are infected by a variety of organisms, and, thus, the obvious issue is cleansing and sterilizing the wound. Here are the crucial steps to take in the event of a puncture wound (or deep laceration):

1. Thoroughly flush the wound with clean water. Use pressure, such as a hose or faucet, to force debris and germs from the wound.

2. If you are helping another individual, never touch the wound with your own hands. Germs from foreign hands are a major cause of life-threatening infections in deep wounds.

3. If there is noticeable debris, such as wood or metal chips, lodged in the wound that fails to dislodge with flushing, attempt the following:

> a) heat a tweezers with fire until the tip turns red hot (be sure to simultaneously protect your hands); let cool.

Then, without allowing the tweezers to touch anything else, attempt to remove the foreign body (this applies to minor wounds only).

Puncture wounds are not hopeless. This is because natural antiseptics can usually salvage the dilemma. After cleansing the wound, use the following antiseptics to halt infection.

Puncture wound combat kit
• oil of oregano — saturate puncture wound site; take 2 or more drops under the tongue twice daily.
• oil of lavender — saturate puncture wound site.
• oil of bay leaf — take 5 drops twice daily.
• raw honey — use as needed.

Radiation poisoning (see also Nuclear catastrophe)
Currently, largely as a result of global governmental instability and aging infrastructure, there is a greater risk than ever before of a massive nuclear catastrophe. The risks of a power plant meltdown have increased largely because of the Y2K computer glitch. Yet, there are other more pervasive ways to develop radiation toxicity besides a nuclear catastrophe or exposure from a nuclear plant. It can happen right in the individual's home: radon. This gas is found in the bedrock of every state in this country. This is a type of natural gassing, where the earth releases radon gases, which are produced as a result of chemical reactions in the earth's greatest nuclear reactor: its molten core.

The only way to determine if you are being exposed to excessive levels is to be tested, that is to have your home tested. Check the local yellow pages for companies offering this service. You may also purchase self-administered test kits.

X-rays are another type of radiation. This is the most common type of human poisoning. Most individuals are poisoned as a result of medical x-rays, which, when performed repeatedly, result in significant tissue damage. X-ray technicians, radiologists, orthopedists, chiropractors, chiropractic assistants, cardiologists, dentists, and dental assistants are highly vulnerable to developing radiation poisoning.

High tension power lines are another type of poisoning. In this case the individual is being poisoned by electromagnetic radiation. Radiation may also emanate from broadcasting centers. Microwave dishes and, particularly, powerful radio towers emit respectively microwaves and radio waves, both of which may enter the body and disrupt the cellular machinery. These forms of radiation are highly significant and may cause a toxicity similar to radiation poisoning. Transformer stations for utilities are perhaps the greatest culprit in this category and their emmisions have been directly linked to a heightened incidence of brain cancer.

Cellular phones are perhaps the most prolific and direct source of electromagnetic wave exposure. Many phones produce potent electromagnetic waves capable of inducing "cellular" damage. The electromagnetic power source is a radio transmitter that produces powerful rays, which are capable of penetrating deep into human tissue, including the brain. There, they will incite the formation of free radicals, which may potentially lead to cancer initiation. Regular use of cellular phones appears to be linked to a heightened incidence of brain cancer. A recent study indicates that frequent cellular phones users are up to four times more likely to develop certain rare brain cancers than non-users. Antioxidants particularly active in protecting brain tissue from cellular phone damage include sage, rosemary, cumin, beta carotene, selenium, vitamin C, and vitamin E. For those who must use a cell phone, daily consumption of these antioxidants is advisable.

Computer terminals emit a significant amount of radiation. All manner of gadgets have been invented to block the radiation. Yet, there is little that can be done about it, and because the radiation must be released, a certain amount of it will be absorbed into the body. However, one significant means of protection is to take natural antioxidants on a daily basis.

Patients undergoing repeated radiation treatments and/or who are subjected to frequent x-rays are being poisoned. X-rays cause tissue damage. They do so by bursting apart human genetic material. Recent studies have determined that radiation therapy offers no significant advantage for decreasing disability or increasing life span. Yet, millions of Americans undergo this therapy yearly. For those undergoing this treatment it is crucial to protect the body from the x-rays' toxic effects plus repair any tissue damage that occurs.

During the 21st century radiation accidents/exposure will occur at increasing frequency. Human error, as well as computer glitches, will cause catastrophic radiation releases. As this book was going to press humanity suffered a monumental nuclear disaster. On September 30th, 1999, as described in the *Chicago Tribune,* an "unbelievable mistake" occurred at a Japanese plutonium plant. Strictly due to human error, the fatal blunder resulted in a monstrous release of radiation. Hundreds, perhaps thousands, were sickened. Cancer incidence will skyrocket. Reports in the U.S. that this is a minor accident are bogus. As plutonium dust is being "wash off" buildings and streets, the press would have us believe that only minor damage was done. Yet, plutonium is so toxic that even a millionth of a gram can kill. The Japanese press is more "consumer friendly" that the U.S. press. If the same type of accident were to occur in the United States, there would probably be an extensive cover-up. Unfortunately, the 21st with be fraught with such incredibly dangerous disasters.

When radiation-induced catastrophes occur, protection may be achieved by taking natural substances and/or antioxidants, which protect the tissues from toxic damage. The following herbs, spices, and nutrients help protect the cells and their nuclei via their potent antioxidant actions:

Radiation poisoning combat kit
• oil of rosemary (edible type in olive oil) — to combat acute radiation toxicity take as much as possible, at least 40 drops daily. As a maintenance take 10 drops twice daily.
• oil of cumin — take as much as possible; no limit.
• oil of sage — take a few drops every hour, internally and/or sublingually. As a maintenance take 5 drops twice daily.
• Juice of Rosemary — drink as much as possible, 6 or more ounces daily. As a maintenance take 2 ounces daily.
• Juice of Oregano — drink as much as possibly, 6 or more ounces daily. As a maintenance take 2 ounces daily.
• red grape powder (Resvitanol) — for acute poisoning take 4 capsules per hour, or take the bulk powder, 1 teaspoon every hour.

• multiple trace mineral supplement (iron-free) — iron increases the toxicity of radiation.
• vitamin E (mixed tocopherols or tocotrienols) — for acute poisoning take 400 I.U. every hour.
• crude natural vitamin C and flavonoids (Flavin-C) — take 3 or more capsules every hour. As a maintenance take 2 or more capsules twice daily.
• beta carotene (as natural crude mixed carotenoids) — take 25,000 I.U. every hour. As a maintenance take 50,000 I.U. daily.
• organic selenium — take 200 or more mcg every few hours for a few days. Selenium is potentially toxic, so after a week or two reduce this amount to 1000 mcg daily. After a month reduce this to a maintenance amount of 400 to 600 mcg daily.
• iodine (as Lugol's solution or potassium iodide) — this is crucial, since radiation releases nearly always include the dissemination of radioactive iodine. This chemical rapidly destroys the thyroid gland, which, as a consequence of its normal tendency, concentrates iodine. Thus, if it concentrates radioactive iodine, it unwittingly destroys itself. The key is to load the blood with natural iodine in order to block the poisonous type.
• iodine as kelp (arsenic-free; PureKelp brand is best) — take 4 or more capsules every hour (this is the safest form of iodine).
• Black seed-plus — take 3 caps every hour or two. As a maintenance take 2 caps twice daily.
• NukeProtect™ (a special formula containing the most essential anti-nuclear ingredients, including kelp, iodine, black seed, and selenium) — during immediate severe danger take 3 or more caps every hour; during moderate danger take 4 caps three times daily; as a maintenance take 2 caps twice daily.
• oil of edible ginger (in extra virgin olive oil) — for fighting nausea and vomiting take a few drops as often as needed.

Foods that help
• Brazil nuts (as a source of selenium)
• cloves, whole
• raw almonds and filberts (rich source of vitamin E)
• dehydrated tomatoes and tomato paste (rich source of the anti-

cancer anti-radiation substance, lycopene)
• cranberry juice concentrate (for flushing radioactive chemicals through the kidneys)
• crude sea salt (or iodized salt if the former is unavailable)
• canned salmon, sardines, and tuna (as a source of natural iodine)
• canned shrimp or squid (a top source of iodine)

Note: the rule with radiation poisoning is to be aggressive. The amount of antioxidants required to protect the body is dependent upon the degree of exposure. If a massive radiation release occurs, be equally massive in the treatment. Double or triple the suggested amounts if necessary. Err in excess, because, without massive protection, the tissues will be destroyed. Barring the remote possibility of allergic intolerance the mentioned items are safe edible substances and can be consumed in huge amounts. The Juices are the ideal agents, because they are quickly absorbed, and the individual will need quick antioxidant power to combat radiation. Protect yourself in every means possible. Radiation poisoning is the most gruesome of all illnesses.

Ringworm

This is caused by a fungus, which attacks the skin and other superficial tissues. The fungus feeds on skin cells. It also feeds on hair and nails. The reason it is called ringworm is that when the organism spreads it makes a ring. However, despite its name there are no worms in this ring, just fungus. Ringworm is another name for athlete's foot and jock itch.

Ringworm is contagious. Humans get it from other humans, and even pets can transmit it. However, the latter can also contract it from humans.

If you develop a lesion which is ring shaped and which is itchy and/or red, it is probably ringworm. The only way to know for sure is to procure a culture. However, in most instances this is unnecessary. The following amounts are ideal for children as well as adults.

Ringworm combat kit
• oil of oregano — rub vigorously on involved region twice daily. Also, take 2 or 3 drops twice daily under the tongue.

- oil of myrtle — rub vigorously on involved region twice daily.
- Oregamax capsules — take 2 or more capsules daily.
- Oil of Bay Berry (very soothing) — rub on the involved region as needed.

Things to avoid
- refined sugar, corn syrup, sweets of all types, pop, etc.
- public gyms and locker rooms
- when walking in public places or using showers in places other than the home, never go barefoot. Wear thongs or shoes.
- don't allow the feet to remain wet (outside of water) for prolonged periods. Whenever the feet become wet, attempt to dry them thoroughly as soon as possible.
- never use another individual's sneakers
- thoroughly dry feet & between toes after every shower/bath

Salmonella

This is perhaps the most feared of all food borne infections. Currently, it is the number one cause of food poisoning outbreaks. The commercial food supply is infested with this dangerous germ. What's more, this pervasive, aggressive germ is resistant to the majority of antibiotics.

Typically, humans contract Salmonella through the gut, that is through eating contaminated food. Once ingested, the organism usually causes diarrhea, which can be violent. Salmonella is an exceptionally destructive bacteria and may infect virtually any organ in the body. However, it has a predilection for infecting the liver and gallbladder, where it causes extensive damage. Apparently, it buries itself in this region in order to evade the immune system.

Outbreaks of salmonella food and beverage poisoning are out of control. Incredibly, according to the CDC there are some 2000 different types of Salmonella that can infect humans. At least 5 million cases of salmonella food/beverage poisoning occur in North America every year, clearly signifying this as one of the most dangerous of all epidemics of the modern era. That means one of every 60 or so individuals contracts this infection yearly, definitively proving this is an epidemic. No one is impervious, nor is seemingly any food. Normally, scientists regard this infection as a poultry or raw egg problem. However, there are numerous other foods which act as reservoirs. In May, 1998, Malt-O-Meal cereal was recalled from dozens of states after it sickened hundreds: the cause was a bizarre sub-type of Salmonella known appropriately as "Agona." Also in 1998 the FDA issued a warning that alfalfa sprouts, as well as radish sprouts, were contaminated with both Salmonella and E. coli. The CDC determined that tens of thousands of individuals have been sickened by the germ contaminated shoots. What is most disconcerting is that the CDC's research proved that despite thorough washing the germs remained, apparently because they are lodged inside the cores of the shoots.

Salmonella combat kit
- oil of oregano (may require the SuperStrength variety) — take a few drops under the tongue several times daily. Take 10 to 20 drops in juice or water several times daily.
- raw honey as an anti-diarrheal (use wild Mediterranean honeys if possible) — take 1/4 cup two or three times daily.
- oil of cumin (to drive the germ out of the liver and gallbladder) — take 10 to 20 drops twice daily.
- oil of cilantro/coriander (activates the liver/gallbladder) — take 10 to 20 drops twice daily.
- LivaClenz — take 10 drops twice daily.

Foods that help
- ginger root
- raw onion, garlic, and green onions
- daikon and black radish

Foods to avoid
- raw eggs and poultry of any kind
- commercial milk products
- processed meats

Scabies

Scabies is caused by a mite, known medically as *Sarcoptes scabei*. The mite is from the same family as dust mites, but it is bigger and specifically infects humans. About the size of a pinhead, it may aggressively invade the skin, causing severe itching and inflammation. Usually, outbreaks occur in individuals with weakened immune systems but, increasingly, outbreaks are striking the healthy population.

Scabies combat kit
• oil of cumin — rub on any involved region as often as needed.
• oil of oregano (SuperStrength variety may be required) — rub on involved region.
• Might at Night™ (proprietary essential oil formula) —rub on involved region(s) as often as needed.
• cloves of raw garlic — crush and place on the bottoms of the feet. Also, crush garlic and apply maceration to scabies region. If irritation occurs, discontinue use.

Foods that help
• Eat as much raw garlic and onions as possible. The stench of the garlic permeates the skin, aiding in the mites' destruction.

Sciatica

This painful and debilitating condition is caused by pressure on the huge sciatic nerve either from disrupted lower lumbar vertebrae or muscular impingement in the pelvis. Sciatica may also be induced by toxic chemical exposure, that is exposure to heavy metals and/or solvents, or alcohol abuse. However, it usually results from sudden injury to the spine, lower back, or hip.

Sciatica combat kit
• oil of oregano — rub the oil over the pain distribution. Also, rub it over the lower back, since this is where the nerve arises. Take 5 to 10 drops twice daily with meals until pain subsides. Take 2 to 4 drops daily in juice or under the tongue as a maintenance.

- red grape powder (Resvitanol) — take 4 capsules three times daily.
- oil of rosemary — take 10 drops twice daily.
- bromelain/papain (BromaZyme) — between meals, take 3 to 5 capsules twice daily.

Foods that help
- fatty fish (salmon and albacore tuna), almonds (high in salycilates), and dried papaya or kiwi (high in enzymes)

Things to avoid
Don't use a heating pad, wet or dry. This will greatly inflame the nerve. If medical care is unavailable, don't use prescription antiinflammatory drugs during a disaster due to potentially life threatening side effects such as internal bleeding. Don't sleep on the back and beware of sleeping on the stomach; this is disastrous for sciatica. *Other ideas:* Keep moving, i.e. stay mobile, but don't jog. Instead, perform brisk walking. Do high step walking, if possible.

Scorpion bites
This is a limited problem for the general population, largely because of geography. Scorpions only inhabit the tropics, Mediterranean, and small tracts of the United States, notably Arizona, Texas, and Southern California. However, if hundreds or thousands of individuals are exposed to the elements in these states, scorpion bites become a significant possibility. In Mexico scorpion bites are a major disaster, causing some 1500 deaths yearly. Not all bites cause death. In fact, bites only rarely cause deaths. Usually, they cause pain—extreme pain. Yet, the type of scorpion found in the southwestern United States is unusually dangerous, offering a potentially lethal strike.

Scorpion bite combat kit
- crushed garlic cloves — apply juice or maceration to the site repeatedly until relief is achieved.
- oil of oregano — apply repeatedly; take 2 or 3 drops under the tongue every hour.

- Bromelain (i.e. BromaZyme) — take 3 or more caps twice daily.

Foods that help
- vinegar — pour it on the bite repeatedly

Seizures

Only medical personnel can properly deal with acute seizures. Thus, the objective is to prevent them from occurring. This is accomplished by properly nourishing the brain and the glands which support brain function, like the adrenal, thyroid, and pituitary glands.

Essential oils are the most effective of all natural anti-seizure remedies. They have direct action upon the brain, because they are transferred to it directly. This is because the oils are volatile, and they gain quick entrance to the human body through inhalation as well as skin absorption. The highly volatile nature of essential oils allows for ready access to the brain, because there is a membrane in the roof of the nose directly connected to it. This membrane, known as the *cribiform plate*, is very thin, and the essential oil vapors pass directly through it. This is why essential oils are so famous for their relaxing actions and their rapid ability to alter mental state. However, skin absorption is also valuable, because once the oils are absorbed through the skin they are quickly trapped by the blood, which transports them to every organ in the body, including the brain.

Seizure combat kit
- oil of lavender — rub on face, buttocks, and soles of feet.
- oil of cilantro — take 5 drops twice daily in juice or water. Also, rub on face and soles of feet.
- oil of oregano — take 2 drops under the tongue once or twice daily. Also, rub on chest, spine, buttocks, and soles of feet.
- Royal Kick — take 4 capsules once or more daily.
- Nutri-Sense drink mix/food fortifier (as a source of crude natural B vitamins for nourishing the nervous system) — take 3 to 6 tablespoons daily in juice or water.

Foods that help
• avocados (rich in natural B_6 and fatty acids)
• fresh red meat (rich in carnitine and electrolytes)
• sardines, salmon, albacore tuna (rich in fish oils and B_6)

Things to avoid
• food dyes and artificial flavorings
• white sugar and chocolate
• MSG and sulfites
• synthetic perfumes
• clothes that require dry cleaning (dry cleaning chemicals damage brain cells)

Shigellosis
Shigellosis is a diarrheal illness caused by the bacteria, *Shigella sonnei*. It is becoming increasingly common as a cause of diarrheal outbreaks. The diarrhea can be severe, bloody, and life-threatening. The most common source is contaminated water, although food may be poisoned by this germ. The germ may contaminate various sites such as public water pipes, reservoirs, ice machines, private wells, and ice cubes. If you are concerned about a facility's water quality, avoid consuming the water as well as the ice.

The CDC notes that, globally, Shigella is the most common cause of bacterial dysentery. Typical symptoms include diarrhea, fever, chills, night sweats, abdominal pain/cramping as well as blood and mucous in the stool.

Shigellosis combat kit
• oil of oregano (SuperStrength may be required) — take 2 or more drops under the tongue several times daily. Also, take 10 or more drops in juice or water as needed.
• oil of cumin — take 10 to 20 drops twice daily.
• onion juice — 1/4 cup twice daily.
• ginger juice — 1/4 cup twice daily. Or, use oil of edible ginger, 5 drops twice daily in juice or water.
• raw honey — 1/4 cup several times daily.
• Black seed-plus — take 2 or more capsules every few hours.

Foods that help
• clear meat broths with garlic and onion

Shingles

As many as 150,000 Americans are afflicted with this disastrous disease every year. The elderly account for the majority of its victims. They are vulnerable, because shingles usually attacks individuals with sluggish or weakened immune systems. Often, it is provoked by severe stress, grief, and the intake of certain drugs, notably cortisone and arthritis medications.

Shingles is caused by a virus of the herpes family. This is the same virus that causes chicken pox. This herpes virus lives in the body, hiding within the nerves. In other words, it is not possible to "catch" shingles. It is not a skin disorder but, rather, is an internal disease which only surfaces in the skin. It is a extremely painful illness, in fact, according to Dr. S.K. Tyring of the University of Texas at Galveston, it is "a medical emergency." When it attacks the nerves, it greatly damages them, often permanently, unless the germ is quickly destroyed.

Usually, shingles develops in the chest around the rib cage. It may also develop in the neck and face, behind the eye (which can lead to blindness), and in the lower back. The pain of shingles is usually excruciating. Often, none of the medical therapies are successful. The individual is left to wraith in agony, often for weeks, perhaps months or years. Natural remedies are part of the answer and often the only answer.

Case history: Mr. C., a young man suffering from a sluggish immune system, saw me during my professorship at the university. He had facial shingles, but this was only the beginning. The virus had infected his optic nerve, the nerve that supplies the eye. Aggressive treatment with natural remedies, which included intravenous doses of vitamin C and pantothenic acid, saved the eye and within two weeks all of the facial lesions were completely healed.

Shingles combat kit
• oil of oregano SuperStrength — apply directly to lesions or pain area. Take 2 drops under the tongue several times daily. Take also 5 to 10 drops twice daily in juice or water.
• Oregamax capsules — take 6 or more capsules daily.
• oil of lavender and/or Oil of Bay Berry — rub on involved region as well as the face and soles of the feet several times daily.
• pantothenic acid (use capsules not pressed tablets) — take 500 mg three times daily.
• premium grade royal jelly (Royal Kick) — take 4 capsules three times daily.
• bromelain — take 3 capsules three or more times daily on an empty stomach.
• I.V. vitamin therapy; see if your doctor can administer this.

Foods that help
• fatty fish (salmon, sardines, tuna, mackerel, etc.)
• beef, lamb, and turkey
• papaya plus the seeds

Things to avoid
• chocolate, definitely and absolutely
• refined sugar and hydrogenated oil
• corn, wheat, rye
• all nuts and seeds, particularly peanuts

Sinus attacks
Effective medical treatment for sinus attacks is lacking in modern medicine. Despite medication, the attacks seemingly continue without mercy. Major causes of this disorder include infection, air pollutants, and food allergy.

Recently, it was discovered that certain essential oil bearing plants, such as oregano, thyme, myrtle, eucalyptus, savory, cumin, and sage, may be useful in reversing respiratory disorders, including sinusitis. The highly orthodox journal, *The Female Patient*, recommends using spices in the kitchen, as well as therapeutically, "to clear out the sinuses." These researchers suggest that the active ingredient in these herbs and spices is a group of compounds found within the essential oils known as phenol. Carvacrol, the active ingredient of wild oregano, is the most biologically active and aggressive of these phenols. Oil of oregano is the richest naturally occurring source of carvacrol and is highly useful as a tonic for the sinuses and respiratory tract. Other herbs useful for sinus disorders include fenugreek, coriander, black seed, bay leaf, horseradish, and cumin. However, wild oregano is the premier herb for the sinuses. In fact, in regards to sinusitis its utility overshadows the need for other herbs, spices, or tonics.

Sinus attack combat kit
• oil of oregano — for best results take it under the tongue. Also, massage the oil over the sinuses; apply a small amount under the nose.
• Oregamax capsules — take 2 or 3 capsules twice daily.
• HerbSorb (as a source of fenugreek, coriander, and black seed) — take 2 or more capsules twice daily.
• oil of bay leaf — rub under nose or in nostril. Also, take 2 drops twice daily under the tongue.
• Black seed-plus — take 2 or more capsules twice daily.
• Juice of oregano – take 1 tablespoon twice daily.

Foods that help
• cayenne and curry powder
• horseradish
• onions, especially green onions
• radishes and turnips

Things to avoid
• milk products, especially butter
• antihistamines, especially nasal sprays
• NutraSweet and sulfites

Skin cancer

This is a current epidemic afflicting primarily fair skinned individuals. The greatest concentration of skin cancers occurs in the United States, Canada, Europe, and Australia.

Prolonged exposure to the sun is the primary cause of skin cancer. The fact is skin cancer, long thought to only develop over a prolonged period, can become instigated suddenly as a result of severe stress and/or extreme sun exposure. However, dietary factors play a significant role, although this issue has never been emphasized sufficiently. Certain civilizations, despite extensive exposure to the sun, have a lower incidence of skin cancer than Americans. These are cultures in which refined foods, particularly the highly refined sugars and vegetable oils, are unknown. In all likelihood it will be eventually proven that diets high in refined vegetable oils greatly increase the risks for skin cancer.

Skin cancer combat kit
• oil of oregano — apply directly to region, and take 5 to 10 drops twice daily (SuperStrength is best)
• oil of cumin — apply directly to region, and take 10 drops or more twice daily.
• Oil of Bay Berry — apply directly to region and surrounding skin. Also, apply to facial skin and other exposed regions preventively.
• oil of rosemary — take 10 to 20 drops twice daily in juice or water.
• red grape powder (rich in the anti-cancer resveratrol) — take 4 capsules three times daily.
• vitamin E, selenium and beta carotene (natural source)

Things to avoid
• constant direct exposure to sunlight. Wear a hat. Don't totally avoid sunlight, but be sure to protect yourself.
• refined vegetable oils

Smoke inhalation (see also Carbon monoxide poisoning)

This is one of the most common causes of human injury during disasters. It is the number one cause of fire related deaths. The inhalation of smoke always causes tissue damage. Massive inhalation may lead to permanent damage and/or death. The agents responsible for this are various hydrocarbons liberated in smoke, which are highly caustic to human cells.

During a fire involving synthetic building materials (or even natural wood) numerous highly toxic compounds are liberated in the smoke, including acetaldehyde, formaldehyde, and cyanide. All of these substances are potent cellular poisons. In the event of smoke inhalation protect your lungs and the rest of your body with agents capable of assisting it in the detoxification of these compounds. In other words, take large amounts of antioxidants.

Smoke inhalation combat kit
- oil of rosemary — take 10 drops every few hours or as necessary.
- oil of oregano — take 2 or 3 drops under the tongue as needed.
- Juice of Oregano — drink an ounce or more as often as needed.
- Juice of Rosemary — drink two or more ounces daily.
- oil of myrtle or Bay Berry — rub on chest and face as needed.
- organic selenium — take 400 to 800 mcg daily.
- vitamin E and beta carotene — take 1600 I.U. and 50,000 I.U. respectively daily.
- folic acid — take 10 mg daily.

Foods that help
- squash, pumpkin, sweet potatoes
- fresh spinach (baby spinach is best), watercress, and parsley

Things to avoid
- cigarette or cigar smoke (1st or 2nd hand)

Snake bites

Compared to the other injuries addressed in this book, snake bites are relatively rare. The basic fact is that if you leave snakes alone, they will leave you alone. The vast majority of snakes are nonvenomous. Even with the venomous types, the bites are rarely fatal. The fact is a greater number of individuals die because of shock or fright than from the snake bites themselves.

Even so, snake bites can be highly destructive, so it is wise to be prepared. This is certainly not a condition to treat by yourself. However, be aware that for thousands of years humanity has relied upon natural remedies for curing venomous bites. Even today these remedies are used, for instance, the application of a garlic concoction to cobra bites by East Indian snake charmers. What follows are a few of the more reliable remedies:

Snake bite combat kit
• raw garlic cloves — crush cloves and apply maceration. Repeat every hour or two or as often as possible.
• oil of oregano — apply liberally. Repeat every hour or two. Take 5 drops of the oil internally every hour. After a few hours, reduce this to 10 drops twice daily until the condition is resolved.
• oil of cumin — for preventing venom-induced liver damage; take 10 drops several times daily until the problem is resolved.
• juice of raw onion — squeeze as much juice into the wound as possible. Drink any remaining juice.
• bromelain (uncoated) — take 3 capsules three or more times daily to reduce swelling and inflammation.

Things to avoid
• Obviously, avoid panic: stay calm. Panic may do more harm than the snake bite. Get medical help as soon as possible.

Sneezing attacks
This is usually caused by allergic reactions. In particular, it is a common consequence of mold sensitivity. There is one reliable remedy: oil of oregano. Combat it by taking 2 or more drops under the tongue as often as necessary to halt the attack. If this doesn't suffice, dilute the oil in olive oil (5 drops in a teaspoon of oil) and drip into the nostrils. Beware: this burns temporarily; the eyes tear and turn bloodshot. However, this dissipates rapidly and there is no harm done to the tissues.

Sore throat

Sore throat is primarily an epidemic afflicting children. Unfortunately, it has become an epidemic among adults as well. It is usually caused by bacterial and/or viral infection. The germs attack the epithelial, that is skin cells, which line the throat, causing inflammation as well as cellular destruction. They also invade and attack the lymph glands, causing swelling and pain.

Most individuals regard strep as the major factor when dealing with sore throat. However, this condition may be caused by a variety of bacteria as well as viruses and fungi. Mold toxins, which are readily disseminated in the air and which may be consumed via poisoned food, may also cause sore throat. In this instance the mold toxins poison the immune system of the throat, causing severe pain and inflammation. Food allergy is yet another cause. Often, a combination of these factors is involved.

Sore throat combat kit
• oil of oregano — take 2 or more drops under the tongue frequently until soreness is gone. Also, gargle with the oil added to salt water. The salt plus oregano oil are synergistic in germ killing.
• Oregamax capsules — take 6 or more capsules daily.
• raw honey (with or without vinegar) — use as a natural antiseptic gargle. Or, eat (literally drink) the honey, 1/4 to 1/2 cup daily.
• Flavin-C (crude natural vitamin C plus flavonoids) — take 3 capsules twice daily.

Foods that help
• onion/garlic/chicken broth
• vinegar and/or salt water gargle
• ginger root tea

Things to avoid
• antihistamines and aspirin
• corn, popcorn, wheat, and rye
• soda pop and caffeinated beverages, including iced tea

Sour mood and/or negativity

There is nothing worse than being burdened by an individual who is constantly negative. This is particularly precarious in a crisis. Negativity and/or moodiness not only is harmful to the perpetrator but it also assaults any bystander. The point is no one can afford to spend time/energy cajoling emotionally deranged adults (or teenagers) during high stress incidents. Halt this negativity with home remedies designed to strengthen the mind, boost mental acuity, erase apathy, and balance the mood. Remember, mental disturbances often originate from physical ailments such as hypoglycemia, adrenal weakness, and/or nutritional deficiency. For instance, a deficiency of thiamine results in depression and/or anxiety as well as mood swings. That is why this substance is known as the "morale vitamin." There are numerous other nutrients which could be deficient (for more information on the significant role of nutritional deficiencies in mental conditions see Dr. Cass Ingram's *Self-Test Nutrition Guide* or the web site, **NutritionTest.com**). Do not always assume bizarre behavior is exclusively due to a psychological problem.

Sour mood combat kit
• Essence of Orange Blossom (helps balance mood and enliven spirits) — drink straight, add to citrus juice, or, preferably, pour into hot tea as an exotic and reviving beverage. Add one or more tablespoons per cup of beverage.
• Essence of Rose Petals — same directions as above.
• premium grade royal jelly (Royal Kick) — take 4 or more capsules every morning before breakfast.
• St. John's wort (wild high flavonoid type is best) — take 2 to 4 capsules with breakfast.
• Juice of Rosemary — add an ounce twice daily in juice or water.
• Nutri-Sense crude rice fractions/polish drink mix (as a completely natural source of thiamine and niacin) — take 3 or more heaping tablespoons in juice, water, or milk once or twice daily.

Things to avoid
• refined sugar and sweets, especially soda pop
• ice cream

Spider bites

A bite by a spider evokes a great deal of fear, but it is mostly overplayed. The only truly fatal spider bites are caused by the notorious and much feared Funnel Web spider of Australia and the Brazilian Wandering spider, the most fatal of all. North American spiders are largely harmless, except black widows and brown recluses. Their bites are only rarely fatal. However, the bites are painful and can cause significant tissue damage. In fact, *Taber's Medical Dictionary* describes black widow bites as being "excruciatingly painful." Brown recluse bites may be less painful, but the results are equally catastrophic. Often, entire chunks of tissue die as a result of the poisonous effects of the venom.

Obviously, if a bite by a venomous creature occurs, get medical help immediately. Yet, the key to minimizing the damage is to apply natural antivenoms to the wound/bite region as soon as possible and also to take natural substances which combat the poisoning. It doesn't matter what type of spider bite there is (usually the individual fails to see the culprit). The treatment remains the same regardless.

Spider bite combat kit

• raw garlic cloves — crush cloves and place a maceration over the wound. Repeat every 4 to 6 hours.
• oil of oregano — apply several drops directly on the region; gently massage into tissues. Take 2 or more drops under the tongue every 15 minutes initially (for up to 2 hours), then 2 drops under the tongue every hour or two until resolved.
• raw honey — place over wound region by itself or with the garlic maceration.

Note: if there is only a sluggish response, take a greater amount of oil of oregano; double or triple the dose. Antivenom is available at hospitals.

Sprained joints

Sprains and strains are widespread in athletically active individuals. Such injuries are a major dilemma in adolescents, especially those involved in aggressive sports.

There are no dependable medical treatments for these injuries. However, natural remedies are a real boon, as they are astonishingly effective when nothing else seems to help. In particular, through the application of oil of oregano, swelling and pain are often eradicated within minutes. The following amounts apply to teenagers and adults. For children reduce the internal amounts by half.

Sprained joint combat kit

• oil of oregano — rub over involved region. Take 5 to 10 drops twice daily in juice or water (SuperStrength is the best for topical application).
• lavender oil — rub on involved region.
• bromelain/papain combination (BromaZyme) — take 3 capsules on an empty stomach three times daily. In the event of a severe sprain double this amount. If the swelling is severe, increase the amount to 5 or more capsules three times daily.
• oil of rosemary — rub on involved region. Also, take 5 to 10 drops twice daily.

Staph infection

Virtually everyone has suffered from some type of staph infection. This hardy bacteria causes boils, pimples, infected ducts/cysts, skin eruptions, psoriasis, sinus infections, sore throats, wound infections, cellulitis, impetigo, and bronchitis, conditions which many Americans suffer with routinely. It is also a major cause of food poisoning.

Staph is also a major perpetrator of life threatening infections such as flesh eating bacteria, bone infection (osteomyelitis), pneumonia, spleen infections, vaginal infections, kidney infections, and blood poisoning. In fact, the commonly feared "red streaks" in the tissues which develop from infected wounds are usually caused by staph infections.

The greatest dilemma with staph is that it has become increasingly resistant to antibiotics. Currently, a bizarre type of mutant staph has been attacking humans, which is immune to all synthetic antibiotics. Known as MRSA (methicillin resistant Staphylococcus aureus) this germ could likely prove fatal in virtually any individual. Deaths from the germ have been reported in Japan, Canada, England, and the United States. It usually attacks hospitalized patients, particularly those undergoing surgery or taking multiple medications. In Canada, where supergerms such as Staph aureus are prolific as the result of the excessive use of antibiotics, massive epidemics are inevitable. Canadian experts predict that as many as 10,000 Canadians will be killed by this germ in the year 2000 alone. Modern medicine offers nothing to stop it.

Now there is a new strain of staph, which is even worse than MRSA. Known as VRSA, this staph is completely immune to antibiotics. The VRSA is even immune to Vancomycin, the most powerful staph killing drug known. According to physicians in the New York region infections by this mutant staph in area hospitals have already reached epidemic proportions. Only natural substances will stop such germs from mercilessly consuming human lives. For instance, according to Cornell University (1998) staph is readily destroyed by natural compounds, including wild oregano oil, for instance, Oreganol capsules, onion, and garlic.

Staph infection combat kit
• oil of oregano— take 2 or 3 drops under the tongue several times daily. Take 10 drops three times daily in juice or water. For tougher conditions use the SuperStrength oil of oregano, 2 to 3 drops under the tongue several times daily plus 10 to 20 drops two or three times daily in juice or water. Rub on any suspect lesion.
• oil of lavender — apply on any lesion and rub on soles of feet.
• oil of myrtle — apply on any lesion as often as necessary.
• Flavin-C — take 6 or more capsules daily to stimulate white blood cell activity against staph.
• Oregamax — take 6 or more capsules daily.
• BromaZyme — take 2 or 3 capsules three times daily.
• red grape powder (Resvitanol) — take 1 teaspoon 3 times daily.
• raw garlic — take as needed, topically or internally

Stomachache

Perhaps the most common ailment of children, stomachaches can afflict virtually anyone. This is one of the most uncomfortable of all illnesses and is often difficult to relieve. This is why natural therapies are so useful, because they offer the ability to quickly abate most stomachaches. The most common causes of stomach - aches include infections, particularly parasitic, anxiety attacks, food allergies, and medication reactions.

Modern research proves that certain herbs aid stomach function. Ironically, many of these herbs, for instance, ginger root, are hot/spicy. This is precisely the opposite of the approach taken by the medical profession, since spicy foods are often prohibited for digestive problems. Yet, in societies where spicy foods are the norm, digestive disorders are relatively rare. What today's medicine has failed to comprehend is that hot tangy spices are tonics, that is they stimulate digestion. Plus, they are antiseptics, which means they kill harmful microbes that cause stomach aches, stomach cramps, diarrhea, and other gastrointestinal ailments.

Stomachache combat kit
• ginger root — slice in hot water and drink several cups daily.
• oil of ginger (olive oil emulsification) — a convenient way to gain the ginger benefits, take 2 or 3 drops twice daily in juice or water. If stomach ache is worse after eating, take oil of ginger with each meal.
• oil of fennel — take 10 to 20 drops twice daily in juice or water.
• Herb-Sorb — take 2 or more capsules three times daily.
• BromaZyme — take 2 or more caps three times daily with meals.

Stomach ulcer

There is a new theory for the cause of stomach ulcers: infection. The culprit is a hideous appearing curve shaped bacteria known as *Helicobacter pylori*. This germ invades the lining of the stomach and duodenum, causing inflammation and, ultimately, ulceration. No one is immune from it. While it is perhaps most common in the elderly, as many as 50% of all children suffering from chronic stomach disorders have the infection.

Nutritional deficiency also plays a role in ulcer formation. Critical nutrients needed to maintain a healthy stomach lining include folic acid, vitamin C, bioflavonoids, vitamin K, vitamin A, thiamine, niacin, vitamin B_{12}, and zinc.

Stomach/duodenal ulcer combat kit

- wild oregano herb (Oregamax capsules) — take 2 or 3 capsules twice daily (plus 2 Oreganol gelcaps for fighting infestation).
- oil of cilantro/coriander — take 5 to 10 drops twice daily in juice or water.
- oil of oregano — take 2 drops under the tongue twice daily.
- oil of ginger (olive oil emulsification) — take 2 or 3 drops with each meal. Mix in juice or add to hot water as a tea with honey.
- crude fenugreek, cumin, black seed capsules (HerbSorb caps) — take 1 or 2 capsules with meals
- Flavin-C — take 2-3 capsules twice daily. In the event of bleeding ulcer, triple this dosage.
- red grape powder (Resvitanol) — take 3 capsules two or three times daily.
- Black seed-plus — take 2 or more capsules with meals.

Things to avoid

- apple juice, soda pop, and caffeinated beverages
- fried foods
- nitrated meats (hot dogs, bologna, salami, etc.)

Strep A

This is the infection that killed Jim Hensen of the Muppets fame. One of the most aggressive and destructive of all germs, strep A is the primary cause of flesh eating bacteria.

Strep A is fiercely attacking Americans. Thousands of individuals are mercilessly killed and/or maimed by it yearly. Recently, (March, 1999) an epidemic of this infection struck some 50 individuals in the Chicago area, killing at least 10. In these instances the germ literally ate the individuals' tissues alive, killing them within 24 to 48 hours. Physicians stood by helplessly, with no cures offered. As the media disseminated the story panic developed, causing thousands of individuals to flood hospitals.

Strep can infect virtually any organ in the body. It is a major cause of drug resistant infections in hospitals and frequently causes post surgical infections. Strep is a primary cause of sore throats, chest infections, heart valve infections, kidney infections, skin infections, tonsillitis, and blood poisoning.

Medicine cannot halt it. Yet, strep A can be destroyed by a wide variety of natural substances, including oil of oregano, oil of lavender, oil of bay leaf, raw garlic, raw onion, raw honey, and cinnamon. Oil of oregano is particularly harmful to this germ. One study found that the oil effectively killed strep by causing its cell walls to disintegrate.

It is automatically assumed that sore throats are due to strep infections, yet, according to *Postgraduate Medicine*, January, 1997, only 10% of teenagers and as few as 40% of children presenting at doctors' offices with sore throats actually have the infection. The other causes, such as viruses, yeasts, and molds, are usually missed.

Strep A combat kit
• oil of oregano (the SuperStrength may be required) — take 2 to 3 drops under the tongue several times daily. Also, take 20 drops in juice or water three or more times daily. Rub on spine and buttocks liberally. For tougher conditions follow the same amounts using the SuperStrength. Or, use Oreganol gelcaps, 1 or 2 caps twice daily.
• oil of lavender (wild mountain grown type is best) — rub on face, chest, soles of feet, and buttocks.
• Oregamax capsules — take a minimum of 3 capsules three times daily.
• Flavin-C (to help activate white blood cells against strep) — take 6 or more capsules daily.
• oil of cinnamon (from edible cinnamon bark, food-grade) — ideal for children, take 2 or more drops twice daily.

Foods that help
• papaya plus the seeds
• raw garlic and onion

Things to avoid
• all forms of refined sugar
• coffee, tea, iced tea, NutraSweet

Sunburn (see also Burns)

Sunburn is one of the most agonizing and noxious of all burn injuries. It's a common human injury, afflicting tens of millions of Americans every year. Every summer millions of Americans develop sunburns severe enough to cause tissue damage.

With modern technology it is possible to prevent sunburns. This is largely through the combination of protective clothing along with sunscreen. While not a magic potion, sunscreen, if used properly, will prevent severe sunburn. The problem is usually that people use too little or apply the wrong type. Light skinned individuals in particular should slather it on. Be sure the sunscreen is guaranteed to block both types of UV light, the A waves and B waves. The best sunscreens use vitamins, as well as antioxidants, as active ingredients. These natural substances are of more value in protecting the skin than merely using chemicals, because the nutrients help heal skin damage. PABA is a B vitamin which absorbs sun rays, preventing them from damaging the skin. Some people are allergic to PABA, so test a small amount before using. Vitamin E, beta carotene, pantothenic acid, and vitamin C also block ultraviolet rays, while helping repair any damage. Ideally, also use sunscreens that have an aloe vera or camomile base, as both of these herbs help induce skin healing.

Certain antioxidant-rich essential oils, particularly spice or herbal oils, act as natural skin protection. This is because such oils, like oils of sage, lavender, and rosemary, are highly potent antioxidants. I have successfully used oil of wild sage and oil of wild rosemary in the Mediterranean to halt sunburn and heal damaged tissue. Simply rub these oils on the body in the morning and at night.

Don't use sunscreens as an excuse to bake yourself. Use them to protect the skin from normal sun exposure. A recent study found that sunscreens may cause individuals to receive damaging sun exposure, because of a failure to experience the benefit of the natural warnings of being burned such as redness, peeling skin, pain, etc. As always, avoid constant direct exposure to the sun. Indirect exposure provides plenty of nourishing sunshine without the damaging effects. Remember, fair skinned individuals have no natural protection against the sun, and they must guard themselves against it. What's more, protective covering, that is the judicious use of hats and other protective clothing, is equally as important as sunscreen in avoiding the damage.

Sunburn combat kit
- aloe vera gel or cream — helps cool skin and speeds healing.
- oil of oregano — aggressive and powerful; prevents scars and halts pain; apply as needed (stops pain and blistering).
- Oil of Bay Berry — soothing/cooling; speeds healing
- oil of lavender — soothing/cooling; speeds healing and is a natural anesthetic.
- BromaZyme — take 2 or more capsules several times daily.
- Oil of wild sage or rosemary — rub topically on exposed parts, morning and evening.

Swimmer's ear (see also ear infections)
This is merely an infection or irritation of the outer ear canal. It is commonly contracted from swimming in germ or parasite infested water. Few people realize that the water in swimming pools, lakes, or seas is readily contaminated with pathogens. When the numbers of these pathogens in natural waters reaches certain levels, swimming is banned. However, even during "legal" swimming periods, a large enough number of pathogenic organisms remain in the water and can cause human diseases. The water-borne pathogens readily infect the outer ear canal. Viruses, bacteria, bacteria-like organisms, fungi, protozoans, amoebas, and parasitic worms can all gain entrance to the body through the ear canal.

Most outer ear infections are caused by bacteria and fungi. The skin of the outer ear offers a moist, nutrient-rich environment, which is precisely what these organisms require for growth. Candida commonly infects the outer ear canal, and usage of antibiotics and/or birth control pills increases the likelihood for the development of this infection. Symptoms depend upon whether the infection is acute or chronic. In acute infection symptoms include pain, aching, and discharge. With chronic infection the symptoms are primarily fullness in the ear, excessive wax, irritation, and itching.

Treatment is simple; application of essential oils on the outer ear and, if necessary, in the ear canal. Do not use full strength aromatherapy oils in the ear canal. Use only the emulsified oils (in olive oil), which are safe for topical application (for instance, oil of oregano, oil of myrtle, or oil of rosemary, etc.). Also, take oil of oregano internally, 2 to 3 drops under the tongue twice daily.

Swimmer's ear combat kit
• oil of oregano — apply about (but not in) the ear or ear lobe. Also, take 2 or more drops under the tongue once or twice daily.
• oil of myrtle — apply on skin behind the ear as an aromatic aid.
• oil of bay leaf — apply on skin behind the ear as an aromatic aid.

Swollen feet and ankles
A number of disorders can cause swelling in the lower extremities, some of which are serious and some harmless. Usually, swelling is a sign of dysfunction of the internal organs. Sluggish function of the kidneys, heart, and/or liver can lead to swelling. Other causes are obesity and food allergy. Parasitic infestation causes swollen extremities, particularly in the legs. One sided swelling in the legs is often due to parasitic infestation, although blood clots could also cause this.

Certain nutrients aid in water mobilization and act as stimulants to normal kidney function. These nutrients include vitamin B_6, potassium, magnesium, and vitamin C. The positive effects of vitamin C are greatly aided by bioflavonoids. Yet, protein deficiency is the most common nutritional factor accounting for swelling in the extremities. This is because proteins are required for the maintenance of normal fluid balance in the body. This is why individuals with this condition often suffer from low blood levels of albumin and globulin, two important fluid regulating proteins. These proteins are produced by the liver. Thus, liver disease may be associated with persistent swelling of the lower extremities.

The Illnesses 267

Swollen feet/ankles combat kit
- oil of fennel — take 10 to 20 drops twice daily in juice or water.
- WildPower Tea (contains natural kidney tonic herbs, wild strawberry leaves and wild borage flowers); drink two cups daily.
- oil of oregano — take 5 to 10 drops twice daily in juice or water. Also, take 2 or 3 drops under the tongue twice daily.
- magnesium chelate — take 600 to 800 mg daily.
- B complex — take 50 mg twice daily.
- Flavin-C (source of crude vitamin C combined with bioflavonoids for strengthening blood and lymph vessels to prevent leaking of fluids) — take 6 or more capsules daily.

Foods that help
- anything rich in protein, specifically eggs, fresh meats, yogurt, whole milk, and fermented soy

Things to avoid
- sugar, sweets, chocolates, soda pop

Tinea capitis (ringworm of the scalp)
A disgusting appearing condition, scalp ringworm is happening in the United States in epidemic proportions. Caused by a fungus known as *Tinea*, this condition afflicts perhaps as many as 1 in 3 Americans. The fact is even simple dandruff is a form of tinea infection. Medical experts proclaim a virtual standstill in curing it. African-American individuals are particularly vulnerable to contracting this infection.

As previously stated the infection in a mild stage occurs in tens of millions and is represented by flaking of the scalp, a type of dandruff. Then, as the infection proceeds the flaking becomes more constant and the flakes larger. Next, the scalp develops a thick scaly layer of red inflamed regions, which may or may not scale. Severe infection is manifested by a ringworm lesion, a well defined round region of the scalp that is tender, swollen, and inflamed. Unless it is promptly treated, hair loss is inevitable. Might at Night is a new formula made from a proprietary blend of natural and wild essential oils. Apply this solution at night as a tonic for improved health of the hair and scalp.

Tinea capitis combat kit
- oil of oregano — rub directly on the site twice daily. Take 5 to 10 drops in juice or water twice daily. Also, add to shampoo for regular use, about 40 drops per eight ounces (or use Whampoo).
- Oil of Bay Berry — rub vigorously into scalp once or twice daily. Leave on for at least 24 hours. Also, try Might at Night.
- oil of rosemary and/or myrtle — rub vigorously into scalp twice daily. Add about 40 drops to 8 ounces of shampoo for regular use.

Tonsillitis

Few parents realize that tonsillitis is a normal consequence of childrens' lives. Children and adolescents contract a multitude of germs and the tonsils are strategically positioned to combat them. That is why they become sore and swollen so frequently. The tonsils are attempting to prevent the germs from gaining entrance to the more significant organs, like the lungs and/or bloodstream.

Germs which commonly cause tonsillitis include strep, staph, viruses, and Candida albicans. It can also be provoked by food allergies as well as allergies to chemicals like sulfites, MSG, food dyes, and artificial sweeteners. The tonsils serve a critical function, since they are a human's first defense at the gate of entry for germs. They should only rarely be removed. Their surgical extraction does compromise immune function.

The tonsils are under constant siege in their attempts to keep the body purified. By strengthening the immune system's ability to destroy germs, the tonsils may be relieved of a great deal of this strain. Thus, they may be retained to serve their valuable role. The following dosages are for children.

Tonsillitis combat kit
- oil of oregano — use as needed, one or two drops under the tongue or in the mouth, usually twice daily.
- wild oregano capsules (Oregamax) — during an attack take 2 capsules every hour. As a preventative take 1 or 2 capsules daily
- raw honey in vinegar — use as a drink to sooth the throat; add water and drink.

• bromelain (as an antiinflammatory) — take 2 capsules three times daily on an empty stomach.
• vitamin C (as crude ascorbic acid with flavonoids) — take 2 capsules every hour until the condition resolves.
Note: the tonsils are fighting a war, trapping and destroying germs before they cause more serious damage (such as pneumonia or blood poisoning). Destroying the tonsils is not the answer. Providing them with strategic support, with added weaponry; this is the most physiological means to utilize. The tonsils exist for specific cause. They should be surgically removed only as a last resort.

Things to avoid
• sweet drinks, especially soda pop
• caffeinated beverages

Toothache
Toothache is usually a sign of infection. If the infection penetrates beyond the enamel, it may enter the root of the tooth, causing severe pain and inflammation. This is known as toothache. The pain is caused by inflammation and pressure on the nerve. This is also known as abscessed tooth. Left untreated, the infection may enter the jaw bone, causing significant illness. Signs and symptoms of a toothache or abscessed tooth include:

• throbbing aching pain in the tooth (or teeth)
• sensitivity of the tooth to cold or hot
• swollen jaw, face, or neck lymph glands
• fever and muscle aches
• tingling sensation in the tooth
• recurrent sinus aches

Oil of oregano is the ideal agent to apply for halting toothache. It possesses monumental pain and germ killing powers. It is also a natural anesthetic.

Toothache combat kit

- oil of oregano — rub the oil on the gums and teeth; saturate a piece of cotton and apply securely against the base of the gum line of the involved tooth; for upper teeth leave overnight. Also, take 2 or more drops under the tongue as often as necessary.
- oil of clove — apply to gums and tooth several times daily.
- oil of edible cinnamon (from 100% edible cinnamon bark) — apply to the involved region as needed (be sure the cinnamon oil is from the edible bark, not the lower root bark, which is unfit for human consumption).

Foods that help

- hot clove bud tea
- wild hot oregano tea

Things to avoid

- refined sugar and sweets, especially soda pop
- chocolate

Trigeminal neuralgia

This extremely painful nerve disorder primarily affects the face. It is usually caused by a virus, which invades the facial nerve, causing extreme pain. The pain is manifested by severe jabs, which shoot like lightning throughout the distribution of the nerve. The pain may be felt all over the face like the tip of the jaw, along the eye, over the forehead, about the lip, etc. The pain is momentary but maddening, as it may repeat itself for hours, even days.

Trigeminal neuralgia combat kit

- oil of oregano (SuperStrength is preferable) — rub topically and take under the tongue, two or more drops three times daily. If possible, rub the oil vigorously into involved region.
- oil of lavender — rub topically and under nose or in nostrils.
- Royal Kick premium grade royal jelly — take 3 capsules three or four times daily.
- oil of rosemary — rub topically as needed and take internally, 5 to 10 drops twice daily.

• Resvitanol (to aid in rebuilding nerve damage) — take 3 or more capsules twice daily.

Tuberculosis

According to *American Family Physician* fully one third of the earth's population is infected with tuberculosis. That makes this disease the number one global epidemic.

In the United States tuberculosis primarily strikes individuals already debilitated by other diseases. However, it is possible that outbreaks of this disease could occur in the general public. What's more, the disease can be disseminated in relatively healthy people through close contact with infected individuals. For instance, several airline attendants became infected when the organism lodged into airline air filters. Passengers are also increasingly being victimized by the potentially highly infectious recirculating air found in airliners. Unfortunately, the airliners have taken no steps to protect the public. Smokers, ex-smokers, and individuals with existing lung disease are the most vulnerable to the development of airline-induced respiratory infections. However, even relatively healthy individuals are falling victim to these infections. Be prepared just in case you are exposed to these unforgiving germs.

Tuberculosis outbreaks will likely occur in the Western world. The epidemics are cyclical, and there is a high likelihood for national or global outbreaks in the near future. Tuberculosis is highly debilitating. The fact is during the early 1900s TB was known as "consumption", because it literally consumed, that is destroyed, the individual. Ideally, the disease should be prevented via the regular application of a healthy diet, plenty of sunshine daily, and the ingestion of potent nutritional supplements. The intake of substances which destroy germs, such as antiseptic spices and herbs (wild oregano is the most powerful), is mandatory.

Tuberculosis combat kit
• Superstrength oil of oregano — take a few drops under the tongue three times daily. Also, take 5 to 10 drops in juice or water three times daily, or take 1 to 3 Oreganol caps three times daily.

- oil of lavender — take 2 drops twice daily in juice. Rub on face, over sinuses, and on chest, also on the soles of the feet.
- oil of bay leaf — take 5 to 10 drops twice daily.
- wild oregano capsules (Oregamax) — take 3 capsules three times daily.
- oil of rosemary — take 5 to 10 drops twice daily.
- Oil of Bay Berry — rub on feet twice daily; also, rub on face and chest often.
- Black seed-plus — take 3 capsules three times daily.

Foods that help
- butternut or other deep yellow squash
- pumpkin soup
- fresh whole milk, particularly goat's milk
- papaya, kiwi, watercress, and chard

Typhoid fever

Now mostly a tropical disease, typhoid fever was once a major cause of epidemics in all parts of the world, including the Americas. The disease is manifested by severe fever, weakness, exhaustion, headache, and abdominal pain. In extreme cases hemorrhaging from the intestines may develop.

Typhoid fever is a bacterial disease caused by a type of salmonella that is carried by various tropical insects. It may also be caught from humans as well as infected milk, food, or water. The most common symptoms are:
- extreme fever with exhaustion
- headache
- abdominal pain
- nosebleeds
- mental confusion/disorientation
- vomiting
- intestinal bleeding (in the extreme)
- stupor, muttering, and delirium

Treatment must be aggressive, since there is a high fatality rate. Much of the treatment should be aimed at detoxification of the liver and gallbladder, since Salmonella aggressively invades these tissues.

Typhoid fever combat kit
• SuperStrength oil of oregano — take under the tongue repeatedly, 2 or 3 drops every hour. Take a few drops in water every 8 hours.
• oil of bay leaf — take 10 drops twice daily.
• oil of lavender — rub on sinus region, face, chest, and soles of feet.
• oil of cumin/cilantro — take 20 or more drops twice daily.
• wild oregano herb (Oregamax capsules) — take 3 or more capsules every few hours.
• Flavin-C — 2 or more capsules every hour.

Foods that help
• vitamin C rich fruit
• great quantities of pure water (add a small amount of salt)
• extra virgin olive oil — consume 1/2 cup daily for at least one week to purge the liver

Things to avoid
• caffeinated beverages
• chocolate and refined sugar

Vaginitis
This distressing condition is one of the most common causes of illness in adult females. Medical treatment for vaginitis is faulty, largely because the condition is usually misdiagnosed. Plus, the treatment, which is broad spectrum antibiotics and cortisone-containing creams, is often futile. This is because in the majority of cases the exact cause is difficult to determine. Plus, the drugs are geared to destroy specific organisms. The fact is there are dozens of germs which may cause vaginitis and most of these germs are immune to antibiotics.

Vaginitis may also be caused by chemicals, particularly synthetic dyes and bleaching agents found in clothes. Lye-based soaps may also instigate the condition. Lye is basic, while the vaginal tract is normally acidic. Thus, soaps, by altering the pH of the delicate vaginal membranes, may weaken local immunity, increasing the risks for infections, particularly yeast infections. Instead of using harsh soaps for vaginal cleansing use pure edible essential oils such as oils of myrtle, lavender, bay berry, and/or rosemary (emulsified in olive oil).

Vaginitis combat kit
• oil of oregano — take 2 drops twice daily under the tongue. Also, take 5 drops twice daily in juice or water.
• oil of myrtle — rub vaginally as often as needed.
• Oil of Bay Berry — rub vaginally as often as needed.
• Oregamax capsules — take 3 capsules twice daily.
• oils of myrtle, lavender, or rosemary — for cleansing and prevention rub on vaginal walls once daily.

Foods that help
• yogurt, quark, and kefir
• sauerkraut

Things to avoid
• refined sugar and chocolate
• synthetic underwear (retains moisture and increases the growth of yeasts)

Varicose veins
This often painful condition afflicts primarily women, the elderly, and the obese. Certain individuals are genetically predisposed to develop it. Varicose veins are caused by the destruction of the valves found inside the veins. The valves are needed to keep the blood moving towards the heart. Without them, the blood backs up, causing congestion, pain, and inflammation. If untreated, varicose veins can lead to potentially serious problems such as varicose ulcers, parasite infections, and blood clots.

Varicose veins combat kit
• oil of oregano — rub on the involved region; take 2 or 3 drops twice daily in juice or water.
• bromelain (uncoated, i.e. BromaZyme) — 3 capsules on an empty stomach twice daily.

• Flavin-C (to rebuild/strengthen the veins) — take 3 or more capsules twice daily.
• red grape powder (rich in natural resveratrol) — take 4 capsules twice daily. Or, take 2 teaspoons daily.

Foods that help
• papaya juice and papaya fruit plus the seeds
• tangerines and grapefruit (eat the inner rind)

Venomous bites (see also Bee stings, Fire ants, Scorpion bites, Snake bites, and Spider bites)

There are hundreds of venomous creatures capable of damaging human beings. However, insect bites are by far the most common cause, with wasps, bees, spiders, and fire ants leading the list.

In the event of a venomous bite there are two essential procedures: 1) don't panic 2) panic enough to seek medical care immediately. Use home remedies as you proceed to receive proper care. They can do no harm and will usually help immensely. The following protocol is universally applicable:

Venomous bite combat kit
• oil of oregano — apply repeatedly, every few minutes, if necessary, plus take a few drops under the tongue several times daily.
• raw garlic cloves — crush and apply juice/maceration on wound.
• raw onion — crush and apply juice/maceration on wound.
• raw honey — cover the wound with it after applying the above remedies.
• LivaClenz (for protecting the liver against poisoning) — take 10 drops three or more times daily.
• oil of cumin (for protecting the liver cells against toxic damage) — take 10 to 20 drops twice daily.
• Flavin-C — take 2 or more capsules several times daily.
• Bromelain (BromaZyme) — 2 or 3 capsules every hour or as needed.

Warts

Warts are caused by a virus known as the human papillomavirus. Wart viruses are inciting epidemics, which remain largely incurable through modern medicine. The wart viruses are difficult to kill and if destroyed superficially, tend to regenerate. Amazingly, there are over 60 different wart viruses.

Wart viruses can grow virtually everywhere but they have a particular propensity for attacking the skin and genitals. They may also invade the mouth, anus, and rectum.

Warts may be a sign of nutritional deficiency, because certain nutrients are required to maintain anti-viral defenses. Nutrient deficiencies which increase the vulnerability to wart infestation include a lack of zinc, selenium, vitamin C, copper, vitamin A, vitamin D, and vitamin B_6. Be sure to take these nutrients on a regular basis.

Few people realize that warts are communicable. If an individual directly touches another person's warts, he/she can develop the infection. According the the editors of *American Family Physician* it is also possible to contract warts from towels, bedding, and other objects. However, the most common way to communicate it is through sex, largely because warts may grow deep inside the vagina, and infected women may not even know they exist. However, they may also hide within the bladder as well as the penile urethra.

Warts combat kit
• oil of oregano (SuperStrength may be required) — take several drops twice daily in juice or water. Also, take 2 or more drops twice daily under the tongue. Saturate a cotton ball or Band-Aid and apply to the involved site; leave for at least 12 hours and repeat.
• oil of bay leaf — apply to the involved site twice daily.
• Oregamax capsules — take 3 or more capsules twice daily.
• oil of myrtle — use preventively during intercourse; also, rub on involved regions as often as necessary.

Things to avoid
• chocolate, soda pop, and refined sugar
• nitrated meats and pork products

Water contamination

Water can either give life, or it can kill. Water related dangers are seemingly infinite in today's civilization. In America alone tens of thousands of individuals become ill from drinking contaminated water each month. The fact is globally there are a greater number of deaths caused from drinking contaminated water than any other factor. Usually, in poor countries bacteria are the waterborne killers. In the United States also bacteria are a major player, but there are other agents of a more insidious nature. Currently, the fresh water in the United States is contaminated by a wide range of toxic chemicals. The public water supply contains thousands of noxious compounds, including heavy metals, chlorinated hydrocarbons (many of which are produced via the chlorination process), pesticides/herbicides, and radiation.

Few people realize that it is legal to dump radioactive wastes into the water channels. Nuclear power plants release untold tons of contaminated water into the sewers and rivers on a daily basis. Hospitals, as well as pharmaceutical houses, legally dispose of radioactive wastes into sewers/rivers. Ultimately, the radioactive poisons enter the public water supply and are delivered right to the tap. Without proper filtration the individual will consume a certain amount of radioactive waste, though it may be immeasurable, on a daily basis.

Humans are mostly water, and, thus, whatever is within the water that people ingest greatly impacts upon health. Incredibly, the entire global water supplies are polluted. The chemical companies know this, yet they continue to produce their dastardly poisons. Plus, it is getting worse daily. A recent study, described in the *Chicago Tribune* (Sept. 12, 1999) and performed by Muhammad Omair, of Ann Arbor, Michigan, provides a vitally important warning. He found that zooplankton, the smallest of all freshwater life forms, are "sprouting growths from their bellies and backs." These growths are essentially bizarre cancers, making up as much as 1/3 of their entire bodies. Zooplankton are a critical link in the food chain and are a clear indicator of what the future bears for humans. According to Omair "the tumors grow incredibly fast." He has discovered them on creatures as young as two weeks. The study was performed using one of the largest bodies of fresh water in the world: Lake Michigan, which supplies water to tens of millions of people living in Illinois, Wisconsin, Indiana, and Michigan.

Why should we care about zooplankton? There should be immense concern, because these creatures are the barometer for future of all other life forms on this planet. In fact, this event is the greatest warning signal of the potential damage caused to humans and the biosphere by toxic chemicals to date. While the Tribune infers a degree of mystery, the cause is simple; dioxin, PCBs, pesticides, herbicides, nuclear radiation, septic water, toxic metals, and similar carcinogenic poisons produced by humankind.

How is this dilemma solved? Certainly, adding a water filter to treat suspect water is perhaps the simplest solution. Currently, in municipalities chlorine and ozone are used to sterilize water. Certain essential oils render water sterile. The most potent of these include oil of oregano, cumin, lemongrass, cinnamon, lavender and bay leaf. Oil of wild oregano was the most effective of these, rendering septic water sterile in a dilution of 1 in 1000. Translated into common terms, this means water can be sterilized by adding 10 drops per cup (8 oz.) of water or about 20 drops per quart. If the water is boiled, much less is needed. For every cup of boiled water add 1 or 2 drops oil of oregano. For every quart add 5 to 10 drops.

A special strength of oil of oregano is available for water or food decontamination, i..e. the SuperStrength oil of oregano. For more information call 1-800-243-5242. This resolves the septic component in a natural fashion.

For everyday protection the use of a water treatment unit may be required. These units utilize modern technological advances, which include activated carbon, to remove a wide range of impurities from the water. Some units also apply sterilization systems such as ultraviolet light. For more information about the state-of-the-art water treatment systems call LifeSource Water Co. at 1-800-992-3997. This unique system removes the vast majority of toxic chemicals. While heavy metals are removed, natural minerals are allowed to pass through. It is a high grade system, superior to the typical type available. Ask for the factory water expert representative. Do call them; your life may depend upon it.

Water contamination combat kit
- filtration straw
- potassium iodide tablets
- oil of oregano (emulsified in extra virgin olive oil)
- pump activated filtration device (military grade)
- chlorine pellets (if nothing else is available; bleach is too dangerous to handle)
- Super Strength oil of oregano (food grade only)

Note: portable water filtration devices are becoming increasingly difficult to procure. This is why natural antiseptics are of such immense importance. Researchers proved that a small amount of oil of oregano, about one drop per two ounces, is sufficient to render fetid water sterile. Always boil suspect water. Then, add a drop of oil of oregano for every one or two ounces. Shake vigorously before drinking. Food grade oil of oregano is available via mail order. To order a vial of pure food grade wild oregano with proven germ-killing powers for water purification call 1-800-243-5242.

Whooping Cough

This was supposedly eradicated as a result of immunizations. Ironically, whooping cough is perhaps the most commonly occurring disease for which children are immunized. Current research indicates the organism may have at best become repressed but, in fact, is alive and infective. This is edified by a recent study published in *JAMA* (August, 1998) and performed in Finland, a country which fully immunizes its population against whooping cough. The researchers found that over one fourth of all individuals with paroxysmal cough have the disease. Astonishingly, virtually all of the infected individuals were immunized. The conclusion of the Finnish doctors is that whooping cough is "common in an immunized population." What an incredible conclusion it is that immunizations offer no guarantee against infection, rather, that despite immunizations the infection strikes thousands. The authors even go so far to proclaim that the value of immunizations for whooping cough (i.e. the DPT) is debatable.

In the United States too the majority of outbreaks of this

disorder occur in immunized populations. The fact is the illness is relatively common in the United States. Researchers have determined that over one fourth of all individuals with paroxysmal (meaning, sudden and spastic) cough have the disease. Thus, the individual must procure alternative means of protection besides the medical approach. The cough may be violent and persistent, scaring parents perhaps even more than the child. The key is to halt the abusive cough and destroy the organism.

Whooping cough combat kit
- oil of oregano — take 2 or 3 drops under the tongue repeatedly until cough stops. Also, take 1 to 3 caps of Oreganol daily.
- oil of myrtle — rub on chest and sinuses, take one or two drops under the tongue twice daily.
- wild oregano capsules (Oregamax) — take 2 capsules several times daily.
- oil of lavender — rub on face, chest, and soles of the feet.
- Essence of Rose — add 1-3 T. in hot water and drink as a tea.
- oil of rosemary — rub on chest or use in diffuser; also, take 5 drops twice daily.
- Black seed-plus — take 1 or 2 capsules three times daily.

Yeast/fungus infection
This is perhaps the number one health catastrophe of modern humanity. Seemingly, it afflicts virtually the entire population of the world, particularly individuals in Western countries.

The high predilection of this germ for individuals in the Western world is largely due to diet and lifestyle. The diet, high in simple sugars and refined starches, greatly enhances the growth of yeasts. Recently, researchers discovered that the consumption of even modest levels of refined sugar leads to a rather massive overgrowth of yeasts. The use of antibiotics, which are prolific in modernized countries, readily induces yeast/fungal infections. In fact, a mere course of antibiotics leads to potentially monumental fungal overgrowth. Just think what is happening to those individuals who routinely use them. They harbor tens of billions of fungi/yeasts, a circumstance which ultimately leads to a wide range of health disorders. Illnesses associated with yeast/fungal overgrowth include chronic fatigue syndrome, fibromyalgia, arthritis, diabetes, lupus, autism, schizophrenia, eczema, psoriasis, cystitis, vaginitis, endometriosis, PMS, seborrhea, Crohn's disease, ulcerative colitis, adrenal insufficiency, hypothyroidism, obstructive lung disease, Sjogren's syndrome, and alcoholism.

In the mid 1970s researchers discovered that when certain spices were added to food the growth of food spoiling molds was halted. In the test tube they found that hot tangy spices were readily able to destroy fungi, even if the spices were used in small quantities. Many individuals regard garlic as the most powerful of all germ killers. Yet, the researchers found that oregano, particularly the wild edible extracted oil, was the most powerful of all germ killing spices. Commercially grown oregano exerts certain antiseptic actions. Yet, the wild high mountain varieties were determined to be even more powerful. Greek researchers, publishing in the *Journal of Agriculture and Food Chemistry* (1995), determined that the wild variety of oregano oil was 400% more powerful than any previously tested. Yet, the most monumental studies of all are being performed currently by Georgetown University (Washington, D. C.). There (1999-2001), researchers are discovering that wild oil of oregano completely obliterates the growth of one of the most difficult to kill of all fungi: Candida albicans. In a concentration of less than a half percent the oil totally decimated all fungal growth. The oil for the research is provided by North American Herb & Spice, because it is from 100% wild high mountain sources.

Nuclear contamination of the earth is causing epidemic fungal infections. The infestation of molds and fungi is caused by bizarre mutant species, which are generated as a result of radioactive exposure. In a study at the University of Iowa a notorious fungus, Candida albicans, was exposed to levels of radiation similar to those from a nuclear accident. Incredibly, not only did the fungus survive the exposure, but it also mutated into some 90 different forms. These mutations are extremely dangerous and can cause frank disease. Thus, the destruction of the biosphere, as well as human health, is largely responsibility of the nuclear industry. The existence of radiation-induced mutants explains the exceptional degree of poor health found in regions near nuclear plants. For instance, it was recently determined that the high incidence of leukemia in individuals living near British nuclear plants is due to bizarre viral infections. While the supposed levels of nuclear irradiation may meet "accepted norms", the mutant germs are insidiously invading living creatures. The so-called clean fuel is destroying the world.

Yeast/fungus infection combat kit
• oil of wild oregano — take 3 or more drops twice daily under the tongue. Also, take 5 to 10 drops twice daily in juice or water.
• wild oregano full herb capsules (Oregamax) — take 3 or more capsules twice daily.
• oil of myrtle (shown by European researchers to be significantly antifungal) — take 5 or more drops twice daily.
• organic selenium (for increasing the capacity of white blood cells to destroy yeasts) — take 400 mcg daily.
• chemical free kelp (i.e. PureKelp) — kelp boosts thyroid function, which increases metabolic rate. Yeasts/molds thrive in individuals with lowered metabolic rate. Take 3 or more capsules daily.
• organic selenium (for increasing the capacity of white blood cells to destroy yeasts; also inactivates nuclear irradiation) — take 400 mcg daily; if exposed to nuclear irradiation, take 800 mcg daily for two weeks, then take 400 mcg daily.
• Fung-E-Clenz (a patented formula containing a special blend of natural spice and herb oils) — to cleanse the body of fungal toxins and residues, take 5 or more drops twice daily.

Foods that help
• garlic, leeks, shallots, onions
• cinnamon and cloves

Things to avoid
• alcoholic beverages, especially beer
• refined sugar
• cortisone and antibiotics
• estrogen and birth control pills
• antacids and H-2 blockers

Yellow fever

According to *JAMA* the occurrence of yellow fever is increasing dramatically. The increase is so frightening that experts regard worldwide epidemics as inevitable. Areas at greatest risk for outbreaks include Africa, South America, Central America, and the southern United States.

Here is the concern. Yellow fever is caused by a virus. The virus is carried by a mosquito, which normally lives in the tropics. However, now this mosquito has adopted urban areas as a residence. In fact, it is found in numerous major American cities, including North American cities such as Miami, Houston, Baton Rouge, and New Orleans. Thus, explosive outbreaks are possible in these cities.

Like dengue and Ebola, yellow fever kills via hemorrhage as well as by destroying the immune system. It takes about 3 to 6 days for an individual to develop symptoms after being bitten. Often, the symptoms are so mild that they are mistaken for the flu, and, thus, no diagnosis is procured. However, a significant percentage become seriously ill. The illness develops over three phases, as follows:

Phase 1: sudden fever, headache, sore aching muscles, nausea, vomiting. Then, it stops for a few hours or up to 24 hours, returning cyclically.

Phase 2: a toxicity may develop, liver damage (represented by yellow jaundice), spitting of blood, dark blood in the stools.

Phase 3: severe high fever, total exhaustion, hemorrhaging, unconsciousness, coma, and death. The latter occurs in 50% or more of those who reach this phase. In children under ten years 8 out of 10 usually die.

In South America significant outbreaks have been reported in Brazil, Peru, Bolivia, Columbia, and Ecuador, with the biggest outbreak occurring in Peru. In Central America outbreaks are reported in virtually every country as well as the Caribbean. In North America there are currently no reported cases, with the last outbreak occurring in New Orleans in 1905, resulting in over a thousand deaths. Yet, the Southern states are long overdue for the return of this cyclical disease. The likelihood of such an outbreak is edified by S. E. Robertson, M. D., and colleagues, who make it clear that yellow fever contaminated mosquitoes have "reinfested" most of the major cities in the deep South.

Remember, yellow fever is a highly dangerous infection. The mortality rate is extremely high. It must be treated aggressively, with emphasis on anti-viral herbs and plenty of fluids. As with all hemorrhagic fevers, major efforts should be applied to strengthen the internal tissues, particularly the blood and lymph vessels, from collapsing and/or degenerating. This means the intake of plenty of bioflavonoids, polyphenols, and vitamin C. The most powerful vitamin C for this purpose is the crude natural type as found in rose hips, acerola, citrus extracts, wild strawberry leaves, etc.

Yellow Fever Combat Kit
• oil of oregano SuperStrength — take 3 drops under the tongue every hour. Take 10 to 20 drops internally several times daily, perhaps as often as every hour if necessary. Imagine this: there are billions of viruses multiplying every hour; so bombard these as aggressively as possible.
• Flavin-C — take 2 or 3 capsules every hour.
• Resvitanol — take 1 t. every hour or 4 to 6 capsules per hour.
• oil of lavender or bay oil — rub all over the face and head. Also, rub on soles of feet, lower back, and buttocks.
• Juice of Oregano — take one or more ounces three times daily.
• zinc chelate — 75 mg daily.
• Oregamax capsules — take 3 capsules three times daily or more often, if necessary.

Foods that help
• Essence of Rose Petals tea (highly aromatic, soothing; helps break fever) or White Coffee (i.e. orange blossom floral essence); drink as often as desired. Prepare by adding 1 or 2 T. in a cup of hot water.
• vitamin C-rich juices
• papaya plus seeds
• onions and garlic

Appendix A
Ordering Information for Nutritional/Herbal Supplements

This appendix lists all supplements mentioned in this book. Many of these supplements are produced by North American Herb & Spice Co. The remainder are manufactured by a variety of other makers. North American Herb & Spice Co. specializes in wild unprocessed natural products rich in original native ingredients. Plus, the label contents are 100% guaranteed to be free of all chemicals, herbicides, pesticides, solvents, or other noxious substances. The products are also unique, because they are primarily from wild plants growing on original native soil. Since the herbs are wild or grown on native soils from natural seeds, which are environmentally protected, there is no possibility of genetic engineering. Thus, products by this company are ideal and dependable ones for any crisis. These products may be ordered at finer health food stores or pharmacies.

Product	Qty	Ingredients
BromaZyme	90 caps	bromelain (from pineapple stems), papain (from green papayas), immature tangerine
Flavin-C, regular	90 caps	rose hip powder, acerola cherry, Rhus coriaria, immature orange, immature tangerine, immature grapefruit, red grape powder
Flavin-C, non-citrus	90 caps	rose hip powder, acerola cherry, Rhus coriaria, wild strawberry leaves, red grape powder
Essence of Orange	12 oz.	orange blossom essence from (white coffee) neroli orange blossoms
Essence of Rose Petals	12 oz.	rose petal essence from Damascene roses
Juice of Oregano	12 oz.	oregano essence from high mountain wild oregano
Juice of Rosemary	12 oz.	rosemary essence from high mountain wild rosemary
Juice of Sage	12 oz.	sage essence from high mountain wild sage
Oil of Lavender	.45 oz.	extra virgin olive oil and wild lavender oil
Oil of Oregano	.45 oz.	extra virgin olive oil and wild oregano oil
Oil of Myrtle	.45 oz.	extra virgin olive oil and wild myrtle oil
Oil of Rosemary	.45 oz.	extra virgin olive oil and wild rosemary oil

Or, products may be purchased via mail order
1-800-243-5242 or via our web site, **wildspice.com**
Guaranteed quality and purity

Product	Qty	Ingredients
HerbSorb	90 caps	fenugreek, cumin, black seed, coriander, and cardamom
Hercules Strength	90 caps	wild rosemary, oregano, and sage
Nutri-Sense	400 g	crude rice bran, polish, flax, lecithin, red sour grape powder, vitamin E
Oil of Bay Berry	1 fl oz.	oils of wild bay berry, myrtle, rosemary
Oil of Cilantro/coriander	.45 fl oz.	extra virgin olive oil, oil of cilantro, oil of coriander
Oil of Cumin	.45 fl oz.	extra virgin olive oil, oil of cumin plus edible fennel oil
Oil of Fennel	.45 fl oz.	extra virgin olive oil and fennel oil
Oil of Sage	.45 fl oz	extra virgin olive oil and wild sage oil
Oregamax capsules	90 caps	wild oregano, Rhus coriaria, garlic, onion
PureKelp	90 caps	wild Northern Pacific kelp and wild Mediterranean oregano
Red grape powder (Resvitanol™)	90 caps	crude unprocessed red sour grape powder
Royal Kick	90 caps	premium high 10-HDA royal jelly pantothenic acid, acerola cherry
Super Strength Oil of Oregano	1 fl oz.	extra virgin olive oil and wild oregano
WildPower Tea	2 oz.	wild strawberry leaves, wild borage flowers, wild hibiscus flowers
Wild St. John's wort	90 caps	wild high flavonoid St. John's wort and wild rosemary
LivaClenz	1 fl oz.	extra virgin olive oil, oils of wild cumin, rosemary, oregano & sage
Oil of Ginger	.45 fl oz.	extra virgin olive oil and ginger oil
Oil of Cinnamon	.45 fl oz.	extra virgin olive oil and cinnamon oil
Juice of Coriander	12 oz.	coriander essence from high mountain wild coriander
Essence of Lavender	12 oz.	lavender essence from high mountain wild lavender
NukeProtect™Oil	1 fl oz.	blend of essential oils
NukeProtect™Caps	90 caps	selenium, iodine, kelp & more
NukeProtect™Juice	12 fl oz.	blend of aromatic essences
Fung-E-Clenz	1 fl oz	blend of essential oils
Might at Night™	1 fl oz.	blend of essential oils (hair and scalp)
Whampoo™	8 fl oz.	cleansing agents & essential oils
Oreganol gelcaps	60 caps	oil of oregano & extra virgin olive oil

Non-edible Emergency and Disaster Items Described in this Text or Recommended for Emergency Protection

portable gas masks and cartridges
protective suits (against radiation/toxic chemicals)
water filtration straws
water filtration units
iodine tablets
geiger counters
diffusers (for volatilizing essential oils)

Specialty mail order food products
"Wilderness Foods"

carob molasses
crude raw wild oregano honey
crude raw orange blossom honey
crude raw wild thistle honey
pomegranate syrup
grape molasses
bulk wild rice
bulk wild oregano
salted jumbo pumpkin seeds
Austrian pumpkinseed oil or ProstaClenz (from NAH&S)
Cooking Oregano
dried high protein foods (beef, turkey, eggs, etc.)

To obtain ordering information call Wilderness Foods at 1-800-243-5242. For an order form or product information send a self-addressed stamped envelope to P.O. Box 4885 Buffalo Grove, IL 60089. These products are grown without chemicals and all are either wild or raised on virgin/native soils. No genetic engineering is allowed. Product quality is guaranteed.

Note: the aforementioned products are of the highest quality, and, thus, are ideal for all age groups, especially children. The quality is related both to the exceptional powers of the raw materials as well as the high standards of manufacturing. Everything is guaranteed.

Supermarket/health food store items mentioned
in this book

canned salmon and tuna
canned sardines
canned herring
canned mackerel

cumin seed
fennel seed
Brazil nuts
peanuts

To procure an ordering/information packet send a self-addressed stamped envelope with four US first class stamps to:

North American Herb & Spice (NAHS)
P.O. Box 4885
Buffalo Grove, IL 60089
To order: 1-800-243-5242
Web site address: wildspice.com

Misc. other products

- selenium chelate (organic selenium)
- zinc chelate
- calcium chelate
- pantothenic acid, 500 mg
- aloe vera
- bee propolis
- lactobacillus
- chlorella

Select Remedies for Specific Conditions

This list is for rapid reference in order to determine the exact remedy needed. It lists the most important remedies, yet there are other substances which may be of immense value recommended within the text. The most important supplements/foods are listed, with the first item being most critical. AIDS, anthrax, nuclear catastrophe, radiation poisoning, and carbon monoxide poisoning require additional critical substances. The following are listed in alphabetically order, like the index of a book.

A

Abdominal pain	oil of oregano, BromaZyme, HerbSorb
Aching feet	oil of oregano, oil of wild lavender, Oil of Bay Berry
Acne	oil of oregano, oil of rosemary, Nutri-Sense
AIDS	oil of oregano, Oregamax, Black seed-plus, Oreganol, Fung-E-Clenz
Allergic reactions	Royal Kick, oil of oregano, BromaZyme
Angina	BromaZyme, oil of rosemary, oil of oregano
Anthrax	oil of oregano, raw garlic/onion, oil of lavender (wild), Oreganol
Arsenic poisoning	selenium, Resvitanol, oil of cumin
Asthma	oil of oregano, oil of rosemary, black seed
Athlete's foot	oil of oregano, Oil of Bay Berry, oil of lavender

B

Back pain	Resvitanol, oil of oregano, BromaZyme
Bed sores	raw honey, oil of oregano, Oil of Bay Berry
Bee stings	oil of oregano, Royal Kick, BromaZyme
Bell's palsy	oil of oregano, Royal Kick, pantothenic acid, BromaZyme
Bites	oil of oregano, Oil of Bay Berry, raw honey
Bladder infection	oil of oregano, cranberry, red grape powder
Bleeding gums	Flavin-C, oil of oregano, Oregamax
Blisters	oil of oregano, oil of lavender, BromaZyme
Blood clots	BromaZyme, oil of oregano, oil of rosemary
Boils	oil of oregano, raw honey, BromaZyme
Bone infection	oil of oregano, Oregamax, BromaZyme
Bronchitis	oil of oregano, oil of wild lavender, Oregamax
Bruises	oil of oregano, BromaZyme, Flavin-C
Burns	oil of oregano, Oil of Bay Berry, oil of lavender

C

Canker sores	oil of oregano, oil of sage, Royal Kick
Carbon monoxide	Juice of Oregano/Rosemary, oil of rosemary, beta carotene, selenium
Cataracts	oil of oregano, Resvitanol, selenium
Chicken pox	oil of oregano, oil of wild lavender, raw honey
Chlorine gas/liquid	oil of rosemary, selenium, Resvitanol
Cholera	oil of oregano, Oregamax, raw honey
Cold exposure	oil of oregano, Royal Kick, PureKelp
Cold sores	oil of oregano, oil of sage, Royal Kick
Colds	oil of oregano, raw honey, Flavin-C
Colic	oil of fennel, oil of oregano, oregano juice
Colitis	oil of fennel, oil of rosemary, Oregamax
Concussion	oil of wild lavender, Flavin-C, wild St. John's wort
Conjunctivitis	oil of oregano, vitamin A drops, oil of myrtle

Constipation	red grape powder, Nutri-Sense, BromaZyme
Cough	oil of wild lavender, oil of oregano, Oregamax
Croup	oil of oregano, Oregamax, oil of myrtle
Cryptosporidium	oil of oregano, Oregamax, raw garlic
Cuts/lacerations	oil of oregano, raw honey, Oil of Bay Berry
Cyanide poisoning	Juice of Oregano, Resvitanol, oil of rosemary

D-E

Dehydration	water, Royal Kick, sea salt
Dengue fever	oil of oregano, Oregamax, raw onion juice
Dermatitis	oil of oregano, Oil of Bay Berry, Oregamax
Diabetes	oil of cumin, HerbSorb, Oil of Cilantro-plus, oil of myrtle
Diaper rash	oil of oregano, oil of myrtle, Oil of Bay Berry
Diarrhea	oil of oregano, raw honey, Oregamax
Diphtheria	oil of oregano, Black seed-plus, Oregamax, Oreganol
Diverticulitis	Oregamax, BromaZyme, oil of rosemary
Dog bites	oil of oregano, BromaZyme, Oil of Bay Berry
Drug overdose/toxicity	oil of cumin, Oil of Cilantro-plus, selenium
Dry or irritated eyes	essential fatty acids, vitamin A, riboflavin
E. coli	oil of oregano, oil of cumin, raw garlic
Earaches/infection	oil of oregano, oil of wild lavender, Oregamax
Ebola	oil of oregano, Oregamax, Resvitanol
Eczema	oil of oregano, Oregamax, Oil of Bay Berry
Ehrlichiosis	oil of oregano, Oregamax, Black seed-plus
Emotional distress	oil of wild lavender, oil of sage, Royal Kick
Emphysema	oil of oregano, oil of rosemary, Oregamax

Encephalitis	oil of oregano, Black seed-plus, Oregamax
Endometriosis	oil of oregano, fish oils/fatty fish, BromaZyme
Exhaustion	Juice of Oregano, Royal Kick, Flavin-C

F-G

Fainting	oil of wild lavender, Oil of Bay Berry, Royal Kick, oil of wild sage, oil of wild myrtle
Fever	oil of oregano, Oregamax, Flavin-C
Fire ants	oil of oregano, oil of lavender, BromaZyme, oil of bay leaf
Flea bites	oil of oregano, raw garlic, oil of lavender
Flesh eating bacteria	oil of oregano, raw honey, raw garlic
Flu	oil of oregano, raw honey, Oregamax
Food poisoning	oil of oregano, raw honey, Black seed-plus
Fractures	BromaZyme, oil of oregano, MCHC
Frostbite	oil of oregano, aloe vera, BromaZyme
Gallbladder attack	oil of cumin, oil of fennel, oil of oregano
Genital Herpes	oil of oregano, Oil of Bay Berry, Flavin-C
Giardiasis	oil of cumin, oil of oregano, Oregamax
Gingivitis	oil of oregano, Flavin-C, Juice of Oregano

H

Head lice	oil of fennel, oil of oregano, Oil of Bay Berry
Headaches	oil of oregano, Royal Kick, Agonex
Heart attack	Oil of Cilantro-plus, Oregamax, oil of rosemary
Heart failure	Juice of Oregano, Oil of Cilantro-plus, coenzyme Q-10
Heat exhaustion	Royal Kick, Flavin-C, sea salt
Heat stroke	Royal Kick, Flavin-C, sea salt
Helicobacter pylori	oil of oregano, oil of cumin, Black seed
Hemorrhoids	BromaZyme, oil of myrtle, Flavin-C
Hepatitis	oil of cumin, oil of oregano, Black seed-plus
Herpes	oil of oregano, oil of myrtle, Flavin-C
Herbicide poisoning	oil of cumin, oil of rosemary, LivaClenz
High blood pressure	Agonex, oil of rosemary, oil of lavender

Hip pain	oil of oregano, BromaZyme, Resvitanol
Histoplasmosis	oil of oregano, oil of rosemary, oil of bay leaf
Hives	Royal Kick, oil of oregano, Oregamax
Hookworm	oil of fennel, oil of cumin, oil of oregano
Hot flashes	Royal Kick, oil of fennel, oil of sage
Hypoglycemia	Royal Kick, HerbSorb, oil of cumin

I

Impetigo	oil of oregano, Oil of Bay Berry, BromaZyme
Ingrown toenail	oil of oregano, oil of wild lavender
Insecticide poisoning	oil of cumin, oil of rosemary, red grape powder
Insomnia	oil of lavender, oil of oregano, oil of sage
Irritable bowel syndrome	oil of fennel, oil of oregano, Oregamax
Itchy skin	oil of oregano, Oil of Bay Berry, oil of myrtle

J-K

Jaundice	oil of cumin, oil of fennel, Juice of Oregano
Jock itch	oil of oregano, oil of myrtle, Oregamax
Joint pain	BromaZyme, oil of oregano, Oregamax
Kidney infection	oil of oregano, oil of fennel, Resvitanol
Kidney stones	Resvitanol, oil of oregano, oil of fennel
Killer bees	oil of oregano, raw garlic, BromaZyme
Knee pain	oil of oregano, BromaZyme, magnesium

L-M

Laryngitis	oil of oregano, Oregamax, Black seed-plus
Lead poisoning	Resvitanol, oil of cumin, Flavin-C
Leg cramps	oil of rosemary, Resvitanol, calcium, magnesium
Lice	oil of fennel, oil of oregano, oil of cumin
Lyme disease	oil of oregano, Oregamax, Resvitanol
Macular degeneration	oil of rosemary, oil of oregano, Resvitanol
Malaria	oil of oregano, Oregamax, Black seed-plus
Measles	oil of oregano, Flavin-C, raw honey
Melanoma	oil of oregano, vitamin E, beta carotene, oil of rosemary, Juice of Oregano
Meningitis	oil of oregano, Flavin-C, BromaZyme

Menstrual bleeding	Flavin-C, BromaZyme, Resvitanol
Menstrual cramps	BromaZyme, Pure-Kelp, oil of oregano
Mercury poisoning	Oil of Cilantro-plus, oil of cumin, selenium
Migraines	oil of oregano, Wild St. John's wort, oil of lavender, Agonex
Mite allergy	oil of oregano, Oregamax, BromaZyme
Mold allergy/reaction	oil of oregano, oil of wild lavender, oil of bay, Oreganol
Mononucleosis	oil of oregano, raw honey, Black seed-plus
Mosquito bites	oil of oregano, Oil of Bay Berry, raw garlic
Muscle soreness/weakness	oil of sage, oil of oregano, BromaZyme

N-O

Nail bed infection	oil of oregano, oil of wild lavender, BromaZyme
Nasal polyps	BromaZyme, vitamin A, oil of oregano
Nausea	oil of fennel, ginger extract, HerbSorb
Nerve gas poisoning	oil of cumin, oil of rosemary, selenium
Nervousness	Wild St. John's wort, oil of wild lavender, oil of rosemary
Nosebleeds	oil of oregano, Flavin-C, Resvitanol
Nuclear catastrophe	Juice of Oregano, Juice of Rosemary, Kelp/iodine, oil of cumin, oil of rosemary, Resvitanol, NukeProtect™, Oil of Bay Berry, oil of sage, selenium, folic acid

P

Pesticide poisoning	LivaClenz, Juice of Oregano, oil of cumin
Pinworms	oil of oregano, oil of cumin, oil of fennel
Plague	oil of oregano, Oregamax, Black seed-plus
Pneumonia	oil of oregano, oil of lavender, Black Seed-plus
Poison ivy/oak/sumac	oil of oregano, tea tree oil (wild), aloe vera
Poor appetite	Nutri-Sense, Oregamax, beef broth
Poor breast milk	oil of fennel, HerbSorb, Nutri-Sense
Postnasal drip	oil of oregano, Oregamax, Juice of Oregano
Prostatitis	Oil of Bay Berry, saw palmetto berry,

	Resvitanol
Psoriasis	oil of oregano, Oil of Bay Berry, Oregamax
Puncture wounds	oil of oregano, oil of lavender, raw honey

Q-R

Radiation burns	oil of oregano, Oil of Bay Berry, selenium
Radiation poisoning	oil of cumin, oil of rosemary, oil of sage, selenium, Resvitanol, Juice of Oregano Oregano, Juice of Rosemary, Black seed-plus, Oregamax, oil of oregano, LivaClenz, NukeProtect
Ringworm	oil of oregano, oil of myrtle, Oil of Bay Berry
Rosacea	oil of oregano, Oregamax, Oil of Bay Berry

S-T

Salmonella	oil of oregano, raw garlic, oil of cumin
Scabies	oil of oregano, raw garlic, oil of cumin
Sciatica	BromaZyme, oil of oregano, Resvitanol
Scorpion bites	oil of oregano, raw garlic, BromaZyme
Seizures	oil of lavender, Oil of Cilantro-plus, Royal Kick
Shigellosis	oil of oregano, raw honey, raw garlic
Shingles	oil of oregano, Oregamax capsules, pantothenic acid
Sinus attacks	oil of oregano, Juice of Oregano, Oregamax
Skin cancer	oil of oregano, Oil of Bay Berry, oil of rosemary
Smoke inhalation	oil of rosemary, Flavin-C, Juice of Oregano
Snake bites	oil of oregano, raw garlic, BromaZyme
Sore throat	oil of oregano, Black seed-plus, Flavin-C
Sour mood/negativity	oil of rosemary, Juice of Rosemary, Royal Kick
Spider bites	oil of oregano, raw garlic, raw honey

Sprained joints	BromaZyme, oil of oregano, Flavin-C
Staph infection	oil of oregano, oil of cumin, Oregamax
Stomachache	BromaZyme, Herb-Sorb, Black seed-plus, oil of ginger (in extra virgin olive oil)
Stomach ulcer	Herb-Sorb, oil of oregano, BromaZyme
Strep infection	oil of oregano, Oregamax, oil of lavender
Sugar cravings	Resvitanol, HerbSorb, oil of oregano
Sunburn	oil of oregano, Oil of Bay Berry, oil of lavender (wild type)
Swimmer's ear	oil of oregano, oil of rosemary, oil of myrtle
Swollen feet/ankles	Resvitanol, BromaZyme, oil of fennel
Tapeworms	oil of oregano (SuperStrength), oil of fennel, oil of cumin
Tinea capitis	oil of oregano, oil of myrtle, selenium
Tonsillitis	oil of oregano, raw honey, Flavin-C
Toothache	oil of oregano, Black seed-plus, BromaZyme
Trigeminal neuralgia	oil of oregano, Black seed-plus, BromaZyme
Tuberculosis	Black seed-plus, oil of oregano, oil of rosemary
Typhoid fever	oil of oregano, Oregamax, oil of lavender

U-Z

Urinary incontinence	Resvitanol, cranberry extract, oil of fennel
Vaginitis	oil of myrtle, oil of oregano, Oil of Bay Berry
Varicose ulcers	oil of oregano, Royal Kick, Oil of Bay Berry
Varicose veins	oil of oregano, Flavin-C, Resvitanol
Venomous bites	oil of oregano, raw garlic, raw onion
Warts	oil of oregano, oil of bay leaf, Oregamax
Water contamination	oil of oregano, oil of bay leaf, iodine
Whooping cough	oil of oregano, oil of rosemary, Black seed-plus
Yellow fever	oil of oregano, Oregamax, Resvitanol

A special message from NAHS, makers of oil of oregano, Oreganol, Juice of Oregano, and Oregamax capsules — oil of oregano and other wild oregano products were introduced to the United States by Dr. Cass Ingram. He discovered the antiseptic powers of the wild herb and crude essential oil in 1995 as a result of a personal illness; oil of oregano had not been in use previously. He then used it successfully to help friends and family. This led to a grass roots movement, wherein the public received immense benefits. Today, oil of oregano, Oreganol caps, and Oregamax caps are among the most sought after dietary supplements known. The discovery will serve humanity forever, since wild oregano is one of the most potent and safe of all natural antiseptics and since few if any natural compounds can match its efficacy. Note that any reference to oil of oregano refers to the high quality mountainous wild oregano produced by NAHS. No responsibililty is taken for those who utilize other or inferior products. The NAHS wild oregano products are guaranteed wild. The quality is also guaranteed, that is your money spent is guaranteed, which is an important consideration and is a reflection of the quality and purity of the product.

A Note by the non-profit Price Pottenger Nutrition Foundation, originated by Weston A. Price, D.D.S.

The Price-Pottenger Nutrition Foundation (PPNF) believes that the full genetic expression of every human being is one of *excellent health, a keen mind, and an attractive physical appearance.* This potential can only be completely expressed when populations consume a diet of *nutrient-rich whole foods.*

The Price-Pottenger Nutrition Foundation *provides guidance for the reversal of modern "civilized" dietary trends that promote disease and physical and mental degeneration.* PPNF provides accurate information on whole foods and proper preparation techniques, soil improvement, pure water, non-toxic dentistry and holistic therapies. This information can help to conquer disease, prevent birth defects, avoid personality disturbances and delinquency, enhance the environment and enable all people to achieve long life and excellent health, now and into the 21st century.

The Price-Pottenger Nutrition Foundation was established as a not-for-profit organization in 1965 to provide the public and the healing professions with historical and anthropological findings and up-to-date, accurate scientific information on nutrition and health. The Foundation is known for its integrity and accuracy in making this information available to the public.

The Foundation is completely independent of commercial interests. Because of its success through the years, it has become heir to the basic research of numbers of other pioneering researchers in the field of nutrition and health.

PPNF serves as a guardian for precious archives and provides access to modern scientific validation of ancestral wisdom on diet, agriculture, life-style, and health. It houses the extensive files, notes and photographs of Dr. Price and Dr. Pottenger, along with the groundbreaking research of William Albrecht, Ph.D., famous soil specialist; Dr. Royal Lee, vitamin researcher; Dr. Edward Howell, enzyme researcher; Dr. Melvin Page, specialist in the relationship between the endocrine system and diet and disease; Dr. Emmanuel Cheraskin, renowned nutrition researcher; and practicing physicians John Myers, M.D. and Henry Bieler, M.D., both known for their success in the treatment of chronic illness.

Our members enjoy reading the PPNF quarterly *Health & Healing Journal;* receiving our free catalog of reprints and pre-reviewed, modern publications; access to PPNF archived material, and our list of healthcare providers. They can rely on the knowledge that the Price-Pottenger Nutrition Foundation serves as a trustworthy source of accurate information on the principles of good nutrition.

We invite you to join us and become a PPNF member. Contact us on our web site at *www.price-pottenger.org* or call us at 1-800-366-3748. Our friendly staff will answer your questions and make sure you receive your membership packet and free catalog. We look forward to hearing from you.

A Note from Dr. Cass Ingram: To all readers, I am a member of this fine organization and am currently an honorary board member. Support this organization for your own nutritional benefit and for the benefit of your loved ones and progeny.

Dr. Cass Ingram's Web Contribution

Soon, an important, monumental web site will become available. This site will assist the individual in determining precisely his/her nutritional needs. Using a highly sophisticated and accurate technology, this system will greatly aid in the correct determination of nutritional deficiencies. The objective is to help the individual rebuild his/her health through accurate nutritional and biochemical assessment. This is followed by extensive corrective recommendations. This is a completely individualized system. It offers two components: dietary analysis and specific tests for a wide range of nutrients. The site will include a monthly Dr. Cass Ingram nutritional update. It is a pay for service site. It is called:

Nutritiontest.com
Test yourself for nutritional deficiencies
**Estimated date of completion: January, 2000. Look it up
on the world wide web**

Notes

Index

A

Abdominal pain, **92-93**, 99, 130, 201, 214, 226, 229, 249, 272, 291

Acetaminophen, 8, 139, 144, 188, 221

Aching feet, **94**, 291

Acidophilus, 143, 144 *see also* Lactobacillus

Acne, 291

Adrenal weakness, 46, 48, **163**, 224, 257, 281

AIDS, 11, 14, **94-95**, 291

Airlines, pesticide use by, 229-230

Air pollution, 94, 101

Allergic dermatitis, **140-141**

Allergic reactions, 61, 73, **95-96**, 101 103, 106, 115, 119, 126, 130, 141, 154, 165, 166, 188, 193, 214, 215, 220, 222, 229, 256, 291

Almonds, 74, 88, 95, 103, 133, 203, 220, 242, 247

Aloe vera, 17, 117, 174, 227, 234, 235, 265, 266

Alzheimer's disease, 41, 49

Amino acids, 35, 66, 72, 74, 77-78, 126

Amnesia, 128

Anemia, 201, 212, 291

Angina, **96-97**, 291

Animal bites, **148-149**, 160

Annals of Internal Medicine, 220

Anthrax, **98**, 291

Apricots, 63, 138, 183

Arsenic poisoning, 32, **99-100**

Arthritis. *See* Joint pain

Artichokes, 142, 152, 185

Aspergillus infection, **100-101**

Aspirin, 8, 93, 139, 140, 155, 169, 170, 188, 219, 222, 256

Asthma, 20, 35, **101-102**, 187, 214, 218, 229, 291

Athlete's foot and/or jock itch, **102-103** 291

Avocados, 133, 175, 180, 227, 237, 248

B

B vitamins, 70, 73, 77, 78, 80, 85, 105, 142, 152, 158, 210, 233, 249

Back pain, 46, **103**, 187, 292

Bad breath, 33, 130

Bay Berry, 105, 109, 113, 117, 120, 132, 133, 134, 141, 144, 145, 149, 156, 160, 161, 167, 171, 192, 194, 208, 227, 233, 238, 243, 251, 253, 254, 265, 268, 272, 274

Bay leaf, 98, 111, 114, 134, 156, 161, 164, 168, 170, 188, 203, 204, 206, 214, 218, 220, 232, 239, 252, 263, 266, 272, 273, 276

Basophilic stippling, 19

Bed sores, **104-105**, 292

Bee propolis, **18-19**, 74

Bee stings, **106-107**, 190, 198, 275, 292 *see also* Killer bees

Bell's palsy, **108-109**, 292

Beta carotene, 44, 55, 69, 70, 84, 85, 120, 160, 210, 211, 240, 243, 253 255, 264

Bible, 24, 37, 67, 68

Bible Hyssop, 37, 40

Bioflavonoids, 111, 116, 151, 159, 163, 183, 224, 262, 267, 283

Bite wounds, **109**, 149, 154, 258

Black seed (Nigella seed), **19-20**, 98 101, 102, 132, 147, 163,177, 178, 221, 222, 227, 233, 234, 237, 242, 249, 252, 253, 263, 272

Notes

Books by Dr. Cass Ingram and Judy Kay Gray, M.S.

#1   How to Eat Right and Live Longer (new edition, Jan., 2000)   **$21.95**
320 pages   6 x 9 inch softback   ISBN 0911119213
Learn to eat right at home, in restaurants, while traveling. This book gives you exact guidance. Learn how to improve your health quickly—just by changing the way you shop, eat, and dine. The food tastes better than ever; includes over 100 recipes.

#2   Self-Test Nutrition Guide   **$29.95**
330 pages   51/2x 81/2 inch hardback   ISBN 0911119507
Everyone is nutritionally deficient. Test yourself for deficiencies from vitamin A to Zinc. Also, test yourself for syndromes such as rapid aging, adrenal burnout, thyroid problems, estrogen imbalance, blood sugar disturbances, parasites, fungus, and liver dysfunction. Corrective recommendations included.

#3   The Cure is in the Cupboard: Oregano for Better Health   **$17.95**
170 pages, 51/2x 81/2 inch softback ISBN 0911119742
Oregano can help you regain your health and then keep you healthy. This is what saved Dr. Ingram's life. Learn how to use oregano and its essential oil for fighting infection and eliminating pain. Combat skin disorders, injuries, wounds, and dental problems. Particularly valuable for fungal infections.

#4   How to Survive Disasters with Natural Medicines   **$13.95**
140 pages   51/2 x 81/2 inch softback   ISBN 0911119442
Honey, vinegar, garlic, onion, papaya, and dozens of other remedies save your life in big or everyday disasters. Combat radiation/toxic chemical exposure, parasitic infection, bacteria, viruses, and water contamination with natural medicines. Specific protocols included.

#5   Tea Tree Oil: the Natural Antiseptic (formerly Killed on Contact)   **$13.95**
125 pages   51/2 x 81/2 softback   ISBN 0911119493
Expanded edition, tea tree oil is a natural antiseptic with unique properties required for anyone's medicine chest. Learn its versatile uses. Information valuable for travelers, wilderness buffs, fishermen, athletes, and parents.

#6   Who Needs Headaches? (How to Reverse Migraines *Naturally*)   **$13.95**
170 pages   6 x 9 inch softback   ISBN 0911119329
Migraines and other chronic headaches are reversible. Find out the main causes (food allergy and hormonal disturbances) and how to correct them. Nutritional recommendations and remedies included; a classic on the subject.

#7   Supermarket Remedies (Power foods for better health)   **$29.95**
330 pages   6 x 9 inch hardback   ISBN 0911119647
Reverse health problems with food, herbs, and spices. Learn about a juice that reverses heart disease and cancer, a vegetable that eliminates depression, a protein-rich food for boosting energy, a berry for improving poor vision, a fruit which lowers cholesterol, a spice that kills germs, plus hundreds of others.

#8   Lifesaving Cures (the most powerful natural cures for the 21st)$19.95
300 pages   6 x 9 inch softback   ISBN 091111999X
It is essential to know lifesaving cures for combating disease, infections, epidemics, crisis, and disaster. Learn how to use dozens of potent remedies for hundreds of illnesses and crises. Global disasters will effect you and they are already occurring: prepare now.

#1 The Survivor's Nutritional Pharmacy—$29.95

Learn exactly how to survive major disasters and everyday injuries that could threaten your health and life. Simple and inexpensive remedies such as honey, garlic, onion, vinegar, and enzymes may save your life. Information different from the book.

#2 How to Use Oregano for Common Illnesses—$9.95

A must addition for oregano lovers. Contains detailed information not found in the book. Specific protocols for dozens of illnesses and diseases plus case histories. Learn hundreds of uses for wild oregano oil and herb—from the Doctor himself.

#3 Wild Oregano: Lifesaving Spice—$9.95

This is the substance that saved Dr. Ingram's life. Wild oregano is the most valuable wild spice of the ancient world, used by Biblical scholars, even the prophets, as a medicinal substance. Discovered by the ancient Greeks wild oregano has been used for germ killing and immune boosting for thousands of years. Dr. Ingram tells his story, the science, and the history behind this amazing compound.

#4 Professional/Advanced Series $89.95*
The Warning Signs of Nutritional Deficiency

4 tapes Total time: 4 hrs   Manual: 100 pages, with Judy Kay Gray, M. S.

Note: discounts available for multiple orders of this series. Ask for information.

Master Dr. Ingram's knowledge about nutritional deficiency and natural medicine. Find out how to discern your specific deficiencies; become proficient in spotting nutritional deficiencies in others. Includes life-saving information on the treatment of disease with nutritional medicine. Become an expert.

* Normal price for this program is $129.95. Save $40.00 when you order from this book.

Shipping Charges: $5.00 for single books—add $1.00 for each additional book. Payment by check, money order, or credit card.

Make checks payable to: Knowledge House
                          P. O. Box 4885
                          Buffalo Grove, Illinois 60089
                          Phone: **(800) 243-5242**

For Visa/Mastercard orders provide the following information:

Card#_____ Exp. Date_____

Signature_____

Name_____

Address_____

City_____ State_____ Zip_____

Order Form

Item	Quantity	Amount
Books by Dr. Cass Ingram and Judy Kay Gray, M.S.		
Book #1 Eat Right and Live Longer	_____	_____
Book #2 Self-Test Nutrition Guide	_____	_____
Book #3 The Cure is in the Cupboard	_____	_____
Book #4 How to Survive Disasters	_____	_____
Book #5 Tea Tree Oil (formerly Killed On Contact)	_____	_____
Book #6 Who Needs Headaches	_____	_____
Book #7 SuperMarket Remedies	_____	_____
Book #8 Lifesaving Cures	_____	_____
Cassette Tapes and Programs		
_____	_____	
Tape #1 Survivor's Nutritional Pharmacy	_____	_____
Tape #2 How to Use Oregano for Common Illnesses	_____	_____
Tape #3 Wild Oregano: Life Saving Spice	_____	_____
Tape #4 Professional Series (*The Warning Signs of Nutritional Deficiency)* (tapes and manual)	_____	_____
Tape #5 SuperMarket Remedies Kit (tapes, video, and book)	_____	_____
Sub-Total		_____
Sales Tax (if any)		_____
Shipping & Handling*		_____
TOTAL		_____

To order call:
1-800-243-5242
Make checks payable to:
Knowledge House P.O. Box 4885
Buffalo Grove, IL 60089

*S & H Charges: $5.00 for single orders - add $1.00 for each additional item. (add $8.95 for SuperMarket Remedies kit). Payment by check, money order, or credit card.